Creating Scientific Concepts

Creating Scientific Concepts

Nancy J. Nersessian

A Bradford Book
The MIT Press
Cambridge, Massachusetts
London, England

First MIT Press paperback edition, 2010
© 2008 Massachusetts Institute of Technology

This book was set in Stone serif and Stone sans by SNP Best-set Typesetter Ltd., Hong Kong.

Library of Congress Cataloging-in-Publication Data

Nersessian, Nancy J.
Creating scientific concepts / Nancy Nersessian.
  p. cm.
Includes bibliographical references and index.
ISBN 978-0-262-14105-5 (hardcover: alk. paper)—978-0-262-51507-8 (paperback)
1. Creative ability in science. 2. Model-based reasoning. 3. Discoveries in science. I. Title.

Q172.5.C74N47 2008
500—dc22   2008013831

In memory of my brother, David Edward Nersessian

Contents

Preface

There are moments of profound insight in science, when, in what seems a blinding flash of conceptual change, the very way we think about the natural world is altered. How do such conceptual innovations arise—what cognitive mechanisms underlie such innovations? This book will argue that, contrary to the popular image of science, such novel concepts do not emerge from the minds of their originators as Athena from the head of Zeus—fully developed and ready to do their intellectual work. Rather, such conceptual innovation, like perfect orchids and flavorful grapes, emerges from lengthy, organic processes, and requires a combination of inherited and environmental conditions to bud and bloom and reach full development.

Very little is understood about the creative thinking that leads to conceptual innovation, and how it achieves its novel outcomes. These creative processes are often thought to be mysterious and unfathomable. Those who study the records of such creations, however, offer a different characterization. Novel concepts arise from attempts to solve specific problems, using the conceptual, analytical, and material resources provided by the cognitive-social-cultural context in which they are created. They are located within "problem situations." So, to understand creativity, it must be located not in the act but in these problem-solving processes. Focusing on the creative act, instead of the process, would be like trying to understand the rainbow by looking carefully at what goes on in a drop of water:

It is not that rainbows aren't made of drops of water, but simply that rainbows don't exist inside drops—they exist only when one takes into account other aspects of the environment of the drop: the direction of a light source, the position of other drops of water, and the position of observers. (Edwin B. Holt, quoted in Reed 1996)

In this spirit, my earlier investigation of conceptual change examined the field concept from Faraday to Einstein, and described the processes

leading to the four major field concepts of that period, including also those
of Maxwell and Lorentz. This analysis showed in detail how each concept
came about through attempts to solve specific problems, and located each
scientist within his problem situation. The focus of that research was the
so-called *problem of incommensurability*, and its associated problem of the
rationality of scientific change. I argued that these philosophical problems
are artifacts of the framing of change, in a way that just compared the
endpoints of a long process, and did not take into account the fine structure in between. For instance, the passage from the Newtonian concepts
to those of relativity theory involved, among others, numerous developments in electromagnetic theory. Many philosophical problems dissolve
when one examines the fine structure of the transitions between theories,
where the various conceptual developments can be seen to be reasoned
responses to particular problem situations.

My investigation of the processes leading up to the field concept high-
lighted another aspect of the creative process—that, in problem solving
leading to conceptual change, the use of analogies, imagistic representations, and thought experiments work hand in hand, first with experimental investigations and then with mathematical analyses. By way of
conclusion—and bolstered by a number of case studies across the sciences
in which these practices are implicated—I hypothesized that rather than
mere aids to thinking, these were powerful forms of reasoning, "model-
based reasoning," and I posed the question of how they accomplish this
intellectual work. That is, how do they generate novel conceptual
representations?

There are many thick descriptions of periods of conceptual change, and
they establish the prevalence of model-based reasoning in such periods.
To borrow a concept from ethnographic analysis, model-based reasoning
transfers across numerous cases from numerous domains. More case studies
will not provide an answer to the question. What is needed instead is an
investigation into the kinds of reasoning that underlie conceptual innovation. That is what I seek to provide in this book.

The nature of creative thought in science has been addressed in history,
philosophy, and the cognitive sciences. Although each of these fields
brings indispensable insights and methods to bear on how the creative
mind works, the fine structure of creative processes is multidimensional,
and explanation requires an interdisciplinary approach, one that uses
methods, analytical tools, concepts, and theories from all these areas. Historical records provide the means to examine the processes and developments of authentic practices, as do ethnographic observations. They record

the development of investigative practices, and provide significant clues as to how novel conceptual developments have come about. Cognitive science investigations aid in aligning these practices with those that non-scientists use to solve problems and make sense of the world, as scientists are not the only ones to solve problems using reasoning strategies such as analogy, imagery, and mental simulation. People involved in mundane problem solving resort to them as well, though not as part of an explicit, well-articulated, and reflective methodology ("metacognitive awareness"). Scientists' use has developed out of these ordinary human cognitive capabilities ("continuum hypothesis"), and thus research into these problem-solving heuristics by the cognitive sciences provides resources to tackle the more elaborate and consciously refined usage by scientists.

The method used in my analysis is thus "cognitive-historical," drawing on cognitive science research to understand the basis of the scientific practices, and reflecting back into cognitive science many considerations that arise in analyzing scientific problem solving. Cognitive science, however, does not provide interpretations and theories that can simply be adopted to explain the scientific practices. By and large it does not study problem solving of the complexity, sophistication, and reflectiveness seen in scientific thinking; thus science provides a novel window on the mind. Further, cognitive processes are most often studied in isolation from one another, such that the research on analogy, imagery, mental modeling, conceptual change, and so forth, are not treated in an integrated fashion. In scientific problem solving, though, these processes are interwoven, making an integrative account imperative. To carry out this investigation of creativity in conceptual change has, thus, required my undertaking an integration of a cross-section of the pertinent research and analysis of foundational issues, as well as advancing new cognitive hypotheses. In achieving all this, the book contributes equally to cognitive science and philosophy of science.

Throughout the analysis offered here I use two problem-solving episodes—one historical (Maxwell) and one think-aloud protocol (S2)—as exemplars of the kinds of reasoning under investigation. For readers familiar with scientific practices in other areas, exemplars from those areas will readily come to mind. Thus, this investigation is not about Maxwell or "S2" per se, but about the kinds of creative reasoning the two cases exemplify. The goal is to understand the dynamic processes of model construction and manipulation as genuine reasoning and as leading up to conceptual innovation. This goal has required shifting the balance of the presentation toward foregrounding the fine structure of the creative modeling processes.

Establishing a cognitive basis for scientific practices, in a way continuous with everyday reasoning practices, does not explain the history of how and why the scientific practices were developed; nor does it explain away the philosophical problems about how they create knowledge. To the contrary, it sheds light on these, and opens new avenues of exploration. Notably, it makes us entertain seriously the possibility that the modeling practices of scientists are not "mere aids," but are in themselves ways of reasoning and understanding that are exploited both in creating and using theories—a core thesis of this book. This project, investigating how models figure in reasoning and facilitate reasoning about phenomena, adds a significant dimension to the growing philosophical literature on models, which largely focuses on the static, representational relations between models and targets.

The objective of the book is to develop a framework for understanding model-based reasoning in conceptual innovation, but the implications of the analysis extend beyond that specific topic. Conceptual innovation is a representational problem—how to represent the known information so as to enable satisfactory inferences that go beyond the target information at hand and lead to novel hypotheses for further investigation. Features of model-based reasoning, as will be shown in the following pages, prove particularly well suited to solving such representational problems.

A growing body of research shows model-based reasoning to be a signature practice of the sciences, and the analysis offered here sheds light on its wider usages within science. For my own research, it stands as a further step in a larger project of investigating how scientists create insights and understandings of nature through modeling—conceptual, physical, computational—and how cognitive, social, and cultural facets of these practices are fused together in scientific knowledge.

Acknowledgments

This book represents the fruits of a long quest that led me to inhabit and learn from communities of historians, philosophers, and cognitive scientists. As such, I have considerable debts to acknowledge, and hope to be forgiven by those I might inadvertently leave out. My greatest intellectual debts are to Lawrence Barsalou, John Clement, Floris Cohen, Catherine Elgin, and James Greeno, who read and commented on either all or chapters of the manuscript (in some cases, several versions). People from whom I have profited in discussing various aspects of the analysis include: Hanne Andersen, Theodore Arabatzis, William Berkson, Susan Carey, Micki Chi, David Craig, Lindley Darden, Fehmi Dogan, Richard Duschl, Dedre Gentner, Ronald Giere, Ashok Goel, David Gooding, Richard Grandy, Todd Griffith, Larry Holmes, Michael Hoffmann, Philip Johnson-Laird, Peter Kjaergaard, Kenneth Knoespel, Janet Kolodner, George Lakoff, Thomas Nickles, Bryan Norton, John Norton, Steven Shapin, Barbara Scholtz, Ross Silberberg, Paul Thagard, Ryan Tweney, Stella Vosniadou, Marianne Wiser, Morton Winston, and Andrea Woody.

Special thanks go to my research group—"the BME gang"—for providing a sounding board for my developing ideas about model-based reasoning and for the many and varied kinds of chocolate with which they sustained me, especially Jim Davies, Ellie Harmon, Elke Kurz-Milcke, Kareen Malone, Wendy Newstetter, Lisa Osbeck, and Christopher Patton. I appreciate the excellent suggestions of Sanjay Chandrasekharan for editing the penultimate version and the assistance of Todd Fennimore in putting the final manuscript into the correct format and tracking down numerous references.

Some sections of this book draw from previously published material: "Model-based Reasoning in Conceptual Change," in *Model-based Reasoning in Scientific Discovery*, edited by L. Magnani, N. J. Nersessian, and P. Thagard, 5–22 (New York: Kluwer Academic/Plenum Publishers, 1999); "The

Cognitive Basis of Model-based Reasoning in Science," in *The Cognitive Basis of Science*, edited by P. Carruthers, S. Stich, and M. Siegal, 133–153 (Cambridge: Cambridge University Press, 2002); "Maxwell and the 'Method of Physical Analogy': Model-based Reasoning, Generic Abstraction, and Conceptual Change," in *Reading Natural Philosophy: Essays in the History and Philosophy of Science and Mathematics*, edited by D. Malament, 129–165 (Lasalle, Ill.: Open Court, 2002); "Abstraction via Generic Modeling in Concept Formation in Science," in *Mind and Society* 3: 129–154 (2003); and "Mental Modeling in Conceptual Change," in *International Handbook of Conceptual Change*, edited by S. Vosniadou (London: Routledge, 2008). I thank the various presses for their permission to republish the material.

I thank Betty Stanton of the MIT Press for persuading me that these ideas needed a book-length treatment and that Bradford Books was the best vehicle for their publication. I appreciate the patience of my editor, Tom Stone, in awaiting the final manuscript. The MIT production staff have been a pleasure to work with, and Judy Feldmann's careful editing has served to improve the book.

I thank the Georgia Institute of Technology for granting me a research leave while finishing the manuscript, especially Sue Rosser of the Ivan Allen College and Aaron Bobick of the School of Interactive Computing. I have profited from several sources of research support over the course of writing. I acknowledge the generous support of the National Endowment for the Humanities and the National Science Foundation, Scholar's Award, from the STS Program (SBE9810913), and research grants from the ROLE Progam of the Division of Research on Learning (REC0106773 and DRL0411825). All opinions expressed in the book are my own and not those of the NEH or the NSF.

Further, I appreciate a fellowship from the Dibner Institute for the History of Science and Technology at MIT where I drafted several chapters, and I thank its former director, Jed Buchwald, and its supportive staff. Finally, I appreciate the Benjamine White Whitney fellowship from the Radcliffe Institute for Advanced Study, which provided the context in which I pulled it all together. Drew Gilpin Faust, Barbara Grosz, Judith Vichniac, and the Institute staff created an amazingly supportive environment in which creativity of all sorts flourished among the fellows.

1   Creativity in Conceptual Change: A Cognitive-Historical Approach

It seems to me that science has a much greater likelihood of being true in the main than any philosophy hitherto advanced (I do not, of course, except my own). In science there are many matters about which people are agreed; in philosophy there are none. Therefore, although each proposition in science may be false, yet we shall be wise to build our philosophy upon science, because the risk of error in philosophy is sure to be greater than in science. If we could hope for certainty in philosophy the matter would be otherwise, but so far as I can see such a hope would be chimerical.

—Bertrand Russell, *Logical Atomism*

Conceptual change is one of the most creative and striking dimensions of scientific practice. Conceptual innovations such as Mendel's notion of gene, Newton's notion of gravity, Maxwell's notion of field, Einstein's notion of space-time, and Watson's and Crick's notion of DNA mark the deep transformations in our understanding of nature, the so-called scientific revolutions. Thus, accounting for conceptual innovation and change is essential to understanding scientific creativity. As such, the disciplines of philosophy, history, and psychology have long-standing interests in studying it, and have gone through periods of mutual influence. The objective of my research for some time now has been to move beyond influence to seek an integrative analysis. The "cognitive-historical" approach provides tools that allow us to explain how scientists often take the first, crucial step in conceptual change: creating scientific concepts.

Discussions of conceptual change have largely faded from the literatures on science in part because the way philosophers framed the problem led to increasingly sterile debates and because the move of historians to more social and cultural accounts of science left the mistaken impression that such facets are at odds with the cognitive dimensions of scientific practice. Over the course of my use and development of the cognitive-historical approach, I have been led to recast the very definition of the problem. I shift the focus from the conceptual structures to the problem-solving practices of the scientists as they change their representations of nature, that is, as they create conceptual structures. Here the practice I undertake examining in fine detail is how models figure in and facilitate reasoning about target phenomena that a scientist seeks to elucidate. One consequence of this shift is to establish a cognitive basis for the scientific practices in ordinary human thinking, while at the same time enriching understanding of cognition in general. Another is the expansion of the notion of reasoning to include "model-based reasoning." Yet another is the demonstration of the contextual nature of problem solving.

1.1   Recasting the Problem of Conceptual Change

Although the "problem of conceptual change" occupied much of the twentieth century, traditional philosophy of science has had hardly anything to say about the central problem of this book: how are scientific concepts created? The problem of conceptual change—and discussion around it— was largely framed by the logical positivists. The problem came to the forefront of concerns in the late nineteenth century, with the development of new concepts such as "energy" and "field," and became of critical importance with the reconceptualizations of physical reality offered by relativity theory and quantum mechanics in the early twentieth century. The development of symbolic and mathematical logic offered philosophers new tools for analyzing scientific knowledge and for attacking the problem of securing the meaning of theoretical concepts in the face of theory change. The logical positivist program for resolving the problem lay in framing it as follows: (1) the conceptual structure of a science can be treated as a language; and (2) the relations of the concepts in these languages to empirical phenomena and to one another can be determined using the methodological tools afforded by logic. Thus, the continuous and cumulative character of scientific change would be established by showing that new or altered concepts are logical extensions of previous notions. Logic afforded the possibility to reformulate—or "rationally reconstruct"—scientific theories and their conceptual structures. These reformulations, not the actual processes of "discovery" of the concepts, were deemed the proper objects of study for philosophers. As Herbert Feigl later stated, "It should be stressed and not merely bashfully admitted that the rational reconstruction of theories is a highly artificial hindsight operation that has little to do with the work of the creative scientist" (Feigl 1970, 13).

The context of discovery traffics in "subjective" factors, such as individual psychology and historical contingency. Rational reconstruction would assure objectivity. Thus, the major work addressing how new concepts are introduced in science, Carl Hempel's classic treatise, *Fundamentals of Concept Formation in Empirical Science* (Hempel 1952), offered techniques amenable to logical analysis for how concepts should be introduced, such as setting up correlations with empirical phenomena via definition and forms of operationalization, rather than treating processes through which current scientific concepts had actually been formed. So, too, Rudolf Carnap in the highly influential essay, "Testability and Meaning" (Carnap 1936), argued that to introduce a new "term" (he preferred "term" over "concept" so as to shed all psychological connotations) into science requires either defining it through antecedently available vocabulary or, for more provisional notions, formulating "reduction sentences" that specify the experimental conditions for its application.

The positivist account of conceptual change remained largely programmatic. Specifying the exact nature of the logical relations among concepts and between concepts and empirical phenomena proved a formidable, ultimately unfulfilled, challenge. Two developments served, finally, to direct philosophical attention away from the project. First, Willard Van Orman (Quine 1951) offered a significant challenge to the central positivist distinction between questions of language (analytic) and questions of fact (synthetic). On his account, there are no epistemic differences between changing one's beliefs and modifying one's conceptual framework. Second, the "historicist" philosophers Norwood Russell Hanson (1956), Paul Feyerabend (1962), and Thomas Kuhn (1962) offered significant challenges. They did so under the influence of Ludwig Wittgenstein's notions of meaning as determined by use and of concepts as forming family resemblance structures rather than definitions. Drawing on their examination of unreconstructed scientific theories and their histories, they claimed that: (1) observation is "theory laden" and thus cannot provide a neutral basis for reduction and comparison for the new and old conceptual structures; and (2) typographically identical terms in the new and old theories, such as "mass," represent "incommensurable" concepts. These claims were bolstered with insights from Gestalt psychology and the emerging cognitive psychology (the "new look" psychology of Jerome Bruner and others). Extensive postpositivist discussion in the historicist vein followed. It centered on the problem of the rationality of *choice* between competing conceptual systems, but largely neglected the prior problem—that of where the new concepts come from.

Most significantly for this book, these critiques also posed methodological challenges. Quine's arguments disputed whether language analysis has
any validity. He advocated "naturalizing" epistemology by using findings
from scientific investigations of humans from biology, psychology, and
sociology to advance the project of justification (see, e.g., Quine 1970).
The historicist analyses demonstrated that the banishment of discovery
and the rational reconstruction approach had led to a conception of scientific knowledge seriously at odds with the practices of science. They
advocated the necessity of history and of psychological and social factors
for addressing philosophical issues about the nature of science.

Whether their arguments and demonstrations were conclusive can be
debated, but the fact remains that the challenges opened up discussion on
methodological questions, specifically: what knowledge is needed to build
an epistemology, and, what methods, other than logical and conceptual
analysis, might philosophers employ in this endeavor? Many philosophers
of science have been availing themselves of an "epistemological naturalist"
response, and my own answers to these questions can be characterized as
a form of such naturalism. That label, however, now encompasses a broad
range of views, not all of which I subscribe to. Broadly characterized, my
research starts from three principles:

1. Philosophical theories of scientific knowledge need to be informed by
the best available scientific understanding of the knowing subject, as developed in the biological, cognitive, and social sciences.
2. Philosophical theories of scientific knowledge need to be informed by
the knowledge-constructing practices used by scientists both over the
history of the development of scientific knowledge and in contemporary
practice.
3. Empirical methods, such as historical analysis, psychological experimentation, ethnography, and computational modeling, can be employed
in developing and testing philosophical hypotheses.

Comparable answers have been given by other naturalist philosophers (e.
g., Giere 1988; Goldman 1986; Kitcher 1993; Laudan 1977; Thagard 1988),
though they differ in the extent to which (1) through (3) play a role in
their analyses. In philosophy of science, the naturalist perspective is a
thoroughly pragmatic philosophy rooted in the study of what scientists
do. This does not mean that a normative epistemology need be abandoned.
Normative recommendations can derive from examining practices that
have borne fruit in scientific investigations and determining, so far as possible, the characteristics that make them successful—if fallible—practices.

As Quine argued, justification and the status of knowledge claims depend on the characteristics of the processes that generate and maintain belief. What I show here through examining the details of exemplars of reflective, creative problem solving that generates conceptual innovations is how each step is based on contextually well-founded assumptions and constitutes a reasonable move.

A naturalist recasting of the problem of conceptual change in science shifts the focus of the problem from the conceptual structures themselves to the nature of the practices employed by human agents in creating, communicating, and replacing scientific representations of a domain. That is, it shifts the focus from the products to the processes, from the structures to the practices. Conceptual changes need to be understood in terms of the people who create and change their representations of nature and the practices they use to do so. To be successful in building an account of conceptual change, thus, requires both a model of the scientist qua human agent and knowledge of the nature of the practices actually used in creating and changing conceptual structures. To address the reformulated problem, I articulated a naturalist method: "cognitive-historical analysis" (Nersessian 1987, 1992a,b, 1995a). How analysis along such lines as I have probed together with a few other cognitive-historical reseachers proceeds will be discussed in the next section. Here one needs only to observe that it creates accounts of scientific knowledge that derive from: (1) empirical data on scientific practices, including their sociocultural contexts; (2) concepts, methods, and analyses from cognitive science; (3) an extensive body of literature on scientific practices in the science studies fields; and (4) philosophical analysis of the problems and issues.

In my earlier study of the development of the field concept from Faraday to Einstein (Nersessian 1984a), I argued that the historical records support the claim that conceptual change is a problem-solving process.[1] Numerous accounts of the history of the sciences beyond my own study provide ample evidence for this position. New conceptual structures do not emerge fully grown from the head of an individual scientist; rather, they are constructed as solutions to specific problems by systematic reasoning. Problem-solving processes are extended in time, dynamic in nature, and embedded in social, cultural, and material contexts. What stands out from this research is that in numerous instances of conceptual innovation across the sciences, the practices of analogy, visually representing, and thought-experimenting are employed. My own investigations center on practices used in physics, but there is an abundance of research across the sciences to support the claim that these practices are especially widespread in addressing conceptual problems.[2] I have taken the ubiquity of these practices to indicate their significance beyond being "mere aids" to thinking in the processes of conceptual change, and cast them, rather, as methods (or "mechanisms") of conceptual change. That is, they are reliable—though fallible—forms of reasoning that generate candidate solutions to representational problems: new concepts. The cognitive-historical method enables its practitioners to tackle the problem of how these practices are productive and, importantly, to do so in the integrative manner required.

1.2   The Cognitive-Historical Method

From a naturalist perspective, addressing the problem of how scientific concepts are created demands a form of philosophical analysis that exploits methods, findings, and interpretations from the history of science and the cognitive sciences. The history of the sciences provides records of the investigative practices through which new concepts have arisen. The historical records, too, enable examining how scientific practices develop. The "historical" dimension of the method, then, investigates the extant records of the scientific practices, examines these over extended periods of time, and locates creative individuals within the problem situations of their local communities and wider cultural contexts. The investigative practices of scientists derive from basic capabilities of the human cognitive apparatus, though of course not only from these. Thus the practitioners of the cognitive-historical method seek to interpret the investigative practices in light of current scientific understanding of what and how human cognitive capacities and limitations could underlie, facilitate, and constrain them. A "continuum hypothesis" underlies the method. The cognitive practices scientists have invented and developed over the course of the history of science are taken to be sophisticated outgrowths of the kinds of cognitive strategies humans employ in coping with their environments and in problem solving of a more ordinary kind. Scientists extend and refine basic cognitive strategies in explicit and critically reflective attempts to devise methods for probing and understanding nature. Studying the science end of the continuum, thus, can lead to deeper understanding of the potential of human cognitive capacities, and contribute to cognitive science research.

The cognitive-historical method is the kind of bootstrapping procedure commonly used in science. The customary range of historical records, notebooks, diaries, correspondence, drafts, publications, and artifacts, such as instruments and physical models, serves as the source of empirical data on the scientific practices. The practices thought to be significant to the objectives of the analysis (in our case, creating concepts) are examined with respect to their cognitive bases. The cognitive science research pertinent to analyzing the scientific practices comprises a wide range of investigations into how humans reason, represent, solve problems, and learn. By means of the cognitive-historical method we consider also in what ways the scientific practices diverge from the mundane findings. Cognitive science is a field under development, and cognitive interpretations and theories are largely uninformed by the cognitive practices of scientists. As with cognitive development in children, the domain of science affords an opportunity to study cognitive processes that involve major changes in representation and understanding. It provides rich exemplars of reasoning in authentic problem-solving situations. Most especially, it provides significant data on metacognitive thinking, as evidenced in the often explicit articulation and reflective refinement of methods, reasoning strategies, and representational issues by scientists.

The cognitive-historical method is, thus, reflexive: studies of scientific cognition feed back into the field of cognitive science, to form the basis of further cognitive research. Studying scientific practices makes a particularly valuable contribution in that their complexity calls for accounts that integrate and unify cognitive phenomena that are customarily treated by separate research areas in cognitive science, such as analogy, imagery, mental modeling, problem solving, reasoning, and decision making. In a cognitive-historical analysis like the present one, the assumptions, methods, and results from both sides are subjected to critical scrutiny, with corrective insights and wider implications moving in both directions. The goal is to bring the practices and the cognitive accounts into a state of "reflective equilibrium" (Goldman 1986).

When addressing the problem of concept formation and change, cognitive-historical analysis strives to understand how it is shaped by the individual, the communal, and the contextual aspects of scientific practice. Although much of the work of creating concepts is carried out by individuals, even when a solitary scientist wrestles with a problem closed in her study or laboratory, she is engaged in a sociocultural process. She is located in a problem situation and uses conceptual, analytical, and material tools deriving from a rich sociocultural context. She is aware that the fruits of her labor will be subjected to the critical scrutiny of her community. But equally, she uses the kind of sophisticated cognition that only rich social, cultural, and material environments can enable. To explain her practices requires invoking cognitive structures and processes. To understand that there is no inherent cognitive–cultural divide and achieve integration requires that each side loosen the grip of the last vestiges of Cartesian dualism (Nersessian 2005).

Contemporary cognitive science offers us one route to breaking free, through reconceptualizing "cognition" by moving the boundaries of representation and processing beyond the individual so as to view scientific thinking as a complex cultural-cognitive system (Nersessian 2006). Those not engaged in or with cognitive science in the last several years continue to identify it with the "rules and representations" or "logicist" account of human cognition associated with GOFAI ("good old-fashioned AI") that initiated the "cognitive revolution." Although much valuable thinking into representation and processing has been provided by that research, contemporary cognitive science is developing alternative accounts and richer, more contextualized studies of human cognition. For nearly thirty years, the traditional cognitive science position has been challenged by research into cognition in real-world environments, and often developed in conjunction with anthropologists and sociologists. As Donald Norman posed the challenge:

the human is a social animal, interacting with others, with the environment and with itself. The core disciplines of cognitive science have tended to ignore these aspects of behavior. The results have been considerable progress on some fronts, but sterility overall, for the organism we are analyzing is conceived as pure intellect, communicating with one another in logical dialog, perceiving, remembering, thinking when appropriate, reasoning its way through well-formed problems that are encountered in the day. Alas the description does not fit actual behavior. (Norman 1981, 266)

"Environmental perspectives" (Nersessian 2005) make human action the focal point for understanding cognition and emphasize that social, cultural, and material environments are integral to cognition. Although not all research from an environmental perspective has taken the system view of cognition, each can be considered as contributing support in its favor. This research comprises the notions that cognition is "embodied" (perception-based accounts of representation such as Barsalou 1999; Glenberg 1997a; Glenberg and Langston 1992; Johnson 1987; Lakoff 1987; Lakoff and Johnson 1998); "encultured" (coevolution of cognition and culture, such as Donald 1991; Nisbett et al. 2001; Shore 1997; Tomasello 1999); "distributed" (stretching across systems of humans and artifacts, such as Hutchins 1995a,b; Lave 1988; Norman 1988; Zhang 1997; Zhang and Norman 1995), or "situated" (located in and arising from interactions within situations, such as Clancey 1997; Greeno 1989, 1998; Lave 1988; Suchman 1987).

Multiple constraints, then, shape cognition. As with mundane cognition, in studying scientific practices "cognition refers not only to universal patterns of information transmission that transpire inside individuals but also to transformations, the forms and functions of which are shared among individuals, social institutions, and historically accumulated artifacts (tools and concepts)" (Resnick et al. 1991, 413). Just as they have constructed physical tools and machines, humans have developed mental "tools" and "machinery" for dealing with and controlling the environment. Science stands at one end of a continuum of such achievements. What distinguishes the development of mental tools from physical tools is that the former develop out of the interaction between two entangled processes: biological selection and adaptation, on one hand, and sociocultural construction, selection, and adaptation, on the other. The epistemic practices of scientists bear both the imprint of human cognitive development and the imprint of the sociocultural histories of the societies in which science developed and continues to be practiced. From this perspective, then, scientific cognition is shaped by the evolutionary history of the human species, by the developmental processes of the human child, and the various sociocultural milieus in which learning and work take place. Scientists extend and refine mundane cognitive practices to meet the objectives of their investigations. Scientific practices can be investigated at different levels of analysis: at the level of researchers as individual, embodied, social, tool-using agents; at the level of groups of such researchers; at the level of the material and conceptual artifacts comprising the context of activities, such as laboratory research; and as various combinations of these.

Placing such scientific practices as I have exhibited here in a case study within the broader framework of human cognitive activities makes it possible to move beyond the specifics of the case to more general conclusions about the nature and function of the scientific practices. In cognitive-historical analyses we use case studies and construct "thick descriptions" of cases (Geertz 1973) as do sociocultural studies, but their objectives differ. The succinct formulation of that objective within cognitive science research by Edwin Hutchins pertains equally to cognitive-historical research: "There are powerful regularities to be described at the level of analysis that transcends the details of the specific domain. It is not possible to discover these regularities without understanding the details of the domain, but the regularities are not about the domain specific details, they are about the nature of cognition in human activity" (quoted in Woods 1997, 177). The "regularities" I am after here have to do with the nature of the interaction of reasoning and representation in conceptual innovation and change. To meet that objective requires identifying the cognitive practices that have led to successful outcomes—outcomes that have advanced science—and then explaining how they are productive, which is the focus of this book. In my earlier investigation of the field concept from Faraday to Einstein (Nersessian 1984a), I described the practices implicated in conceptual change for four major participants in the development of a "field" concept, located each within his problem situation, and discussed the relations among these concepts and how best to represent these continuous but noncumulative concepts. The project of this book is different. The objective is to understand the nature of model-based reasoning as productive of conceptual innovation, and in creative problem solving in general. The analysis begins with two exemplars of the kinds of reasoning under investigation. These provide content on which to hang the analytical framework as it is developed. One analyzes a problem-solving episode of Maxwell, specifying in detail the constraints used in each phase of model construction, manipulation, evaluation, and adaptation, as the reasoning led to his reconceptualization of electromagnetism. The other analyzes a problem-solving protocol in which model-based reasoning that parallels Maxwell's to a significant extent was used by the experimental participant and led to his revising his concept of "spring." The exemplars are developed in fine detail and show how incremental modeling processes enabled each reasoner to use the limited resources at his disposal to overcome conceptual barriers. Juxtaposing these two exemplars also serves to elicit commonalities between creative reasoning in science and in more ordinary circumstances. Because the objective of the present analysis is to develop an account of model-based reasoning and how it is generative of conceptual change, the step-by-step reasoning processes are foregrounded, while the rich sociocultural facets of the Maxwell case, in particular, are provided in outline. Nevertheless, these remain central to understanding aspects of the modeling.

1.3   Reasoning

A wide range of studies lends credence to the idea that model construction, manipulation, evaluation, and adaptation are a primary means through which scientists create new conceptual representations. These findings are in line with an extensive contemporary literature that establishes various kinds of modeling to be a *signature* feature of much research in the sciences: in discovery, pursuit, and application. Many philosophers now agree that the basic units for scientists in working with theories are most often not axiomatic systems or propositional networks, but models (see, e.g., Cartwright 1983; Darden 1991; Giere 1988; Hesse 1963; Magnani, Nersessian, and Thagard 1999; Morgan and Morrison 1999). Histories of the sciences show that in building a theory, modeling often comes first, with further abstraction to formal expression in laws and axioms of theories following. In contrast with much of the modeling literature, I am not primarily concerned with the representational relations between models and targets and other issues of realism; rather, my concern is with *how models figure in and facilitate reasoning about target phenomena.*

Embracing the notion that the modeling practices constitute genuine reasoning has required that I expand philosophical notions of reasoning. Creative model-based reasoning cannot be applied as a simple recipe, is not always productive of solutions, and even its most exemplary usages can lead to incorrect solutions. To countenance these practices as reasoning I have consequently needed to challenge the deeply ingrained philosophical notion that equates reasoning with logic. Although it might be possible to *rederive* the outcomes of a model-based reasoning process by means of logic, that move can take place only *after* the creative work has been done, and so leaves the discovery and creativity processes a mystery. I agree with philosophers of such diverse positions as Reichenbach and Popper that there is no "logic of discovery" (at least no *classical* logic), but I disagree with equating reasoning with logic. The notions of reasoning with which philosophy has been operating are too narrowly constrained and have led to the mistaken view that discoveries cannot derive from reasoned processes.

Traditional philosophical accounts of scientific reasoning construe it as logic-based: applying deductive or inductive algorithms to sets of propositions. Deductive reasoning provides the gold standard, with the essential notion being soundness: true premises plus good reasoning yield true conclusions. Much of scientific practice does not fit that standard. The "hypothetico-deductive" method, which comprises hypothesis generation and the testing of deductive consequences of these, is a variation that focuses the fallibility of science with respect to the premises. This leaves out of the account the prior inferential work that generates the hypotheses. Logical positivism emphasized the inductive nature of scientific inference and tried to develop a notion of soundness for induction. Loosely construed, as by current Bayesian accounts, starting from maximally probable premises and using correct inductive logic one should arrive at maximally probable conclusions. What remains a mystery is how the prior probabilities of a premise or hypothesis are to be determined.

Creative inference is often labeled "abduction," but the nature of the inferential processes of abductive reasoning remains largely unspecified. Formulating an account of model-based reasoning provides a means of specifying the nature of the ampliative reasoning in abductive inference, for instance, analogy.[3] It stands also to contribute to accounts of inductive inference by providing a basis from which to assign prior probabilities; for instance, high prior probabilities might be assigned to hypotheses that result from good analogical reasoning, such as Maxwell's hypothesis that electromagnetic waves propagate at the speed of light.[4]

In model-based reasoning, inferences are made by means of creating models and manipulating, adapting, and evaluating them. A model, for my present purposes, can be characterized loosely as a representation of a system with interactive parts and with representations of those interactions. Model-based reasoning can be performed through the use of conceptual, physical, mathematical, and computational models, or combinations of these. Here I treat conceptual models. These are imaginary systems designed to be structural, functional, or behavioral analogues of target phenomena. The models are dynamical in that future states can be determined through mentally simulating the model. Analogical, visual, and simulative modeling are used widely in ordinary and in scientific problem solving, ranging from mundane to highly creative usage. On a cognitive-historical account, these uses are not different in kind, but lie on a continuum. Studying one end of the spectrum will illuminate the other, but a deep understanding requires examining the range. In creative, scientific usage, we see, for instance, that different representational modalities are often exploited in a single problem-solving episode. Thus my historical exemplar details how Maxwell created visual representations of imaginary analogical models representing aspects of a new conceptual system—the "electromagnetic field." These models were conceived as dynamic—to be thought of as animated in time—and the visual representations of these are accompanied by text instructing the reader how to animate them mentally. Reasoning by means of model construction and manipulation, he derived mathematical equations, theoretical hypotheses, and experimental predictions. I contend that in coming to understand how his model-based reasoning led to a genuinely novel scientific representation, we understand something about the intellectual work that is accomplished through model-based reasoning across the spectrum.

1.4 Model-based Reasoning Exemplars

To recap thus far, the focus of this book is specific modeling practices that historical records implicate in problem solving leading to conceptual innovation, specifically, analogical modeling, visual modeling, and thought-experimenting. I am not claiming that they are the only means of conceptual innovation—just that they seem especially productive means. These practices have long captured the attention of students of creativity in science, and so the literature describing instances is extensive. Another case study is not what is needed; neither is a survey of numerous cases. Rather, I seek to develop an analytical framework for understanding how they are generative. So, instead, I examine in detail two exemplars—each working through the fine structure of an extended problem-solving process with attention to precisely how model construction, manipulation, evaluation, and adaptation work to achieve a plausible solution to the target problem.

Maxwell's model-based reasoning in creating a mathematical representation of the electromagnetic field concept serves as the primary exemplar. This kind of creative reasoning in science is my target. The strategy of concentrating on an in-depth analysis of one exemplar arises from several considerations. First, as a practical issue, analyzing such problem-solving episodes requires a substantial range and depth of knowledge about the subject matter, the problem situation, and the scientist's practices. As with many things, the devil is in the details, and the details are difficult, but to understand the reasoning requires developing them. Second, as is often the case in science itself, the data supplied by one fertile case can provide significant insights into the phenomena under investigation and lead to substantial progress in the research program of explaining those phenomena. Third, in conjoining the analysis with a range of cognitive science investigations, I use the cognitive-historical method as a basis for transferring some major conclusions drawn from one exemplar across a range of of others.

The Maxwell exemplar develops the reasoning in the 1861–1862 analysis in which he first derived the mathematical representation of the electromagnetic field (Maxwell 1861–1862). To what extent can we consider Maxwell's paper to provide data about his actual problem-solving practices? Clearly all published papers are reconstructed accounts intended for communication, explanation, and justification of previously derived results. As such, these are for the most part assumed to convey the results of prior problem solving and not as providing a concurrent record. But even concurrent records present a problem for their interpreters. All historical records are reconstructions by their authors to greater or lesser degrees. Any assumption of total veracity or completeness is underdetermined by the evidence available in the historical record. The best an interpreter can do is use whatever variety of resources are available to construct an argument for the particular interpretation of a case. In Maxwell's case, there is supporting evidence to be found in his correspondence with his friend and teacher William Thompson (Larmor 1937) about his thinking during his problem solving and near the time of writing the paper; in some draft material (though most of Maxwell's drafts were destroyed in a fire) (Harman [Heimann] 1990, 1995); and in comments he made in the papers on electromagnetism and on many other occasions about the fertility of analogy and visualization in solving physical problems (see, e.g., Campbell and Garnett 1969; Larmor 1937; Harman [Heimann] 1990, 1995; Maxwell 1856).

Additionally, as F. L. Holmes (1990) has pointed out, narrative and argument are intertwined in research papers—and this is especially so in nineteenth-century scientific writing. The narrative usually provides a synopsis of the problem solving that is close to the original work in time, and we know from biographical details that Maxwell was writing the paper close to the time of its publication. In fact, the last two parts of the paper did not appear until nine months after the first two parts, because he had not worked out the key problem of representing electrostatic induction at the time of their publication. It is also reasonable to assume that given the spectacular novelty of Maxwell's results, he would attempt to convey them in a way that he found meaningful and that he thought would contribute to his community's understanding both of the results and of how he had achieved them. That is, the intent of his paper is not only to justify his results, but also to lead others to understand the novel representation of electric and magnetic forces as continuous actions rather than actions at a distance and to understand his methodological approach of "physical analogy." Such considerations have led me to construe Maxwell as presenting his research along a path close to his original thoughts. Thus, the paper is treated as presenting a reasonably reliable and highly salient trace through the problem-solving path along which Maxwell derived the field equations.

Both the interest of and the difficulty with using the Maxwell exemplar is its technical complexity. Since this book is intended for an audience that cuts across cognitive science and science and technology studies, I present the analysis in qualitative terms. For the technical details of how the specific equations he derived relate to the models, I refer readers to Nersessian (2002a). However, the Maxwell exemplar is quite complex conceptually, and even the qualitative presentation might prove daunting to readers not familiar with the physics. In chapter 3, I develop a second, less technically complex exemplar that has many of the features of the Maxwell case. This is in the form of a think-aloud protocol of an experimental participant, "S2," solving a problem related to springs that leads to change in his concept of spring. It is an interesting case of conceptual innovation in its own right, and serves two purposes here: first, as a more accessible exemplar of model-based reasoning in conceptual change and, second, as an exemplar of the continuum hypothesis.

And indeed it turns out that the protocol provides substance to the premise underlying cognitive-historical analysis: scientific and "ordinary" problem solving are not different in kind but lie along a continuum. The entire protocol study involved eleven scientists from various disciplines trying to solve a novel but rather mundane problem about springs. The particular S2 case was chosen because it exhibits problem-solving practices in conceptual innovation similar to those used in the historical case. Of course, the significance of the innovations is vastly greater in the one case than in the other. Maxwell created a new mode of representation in physics, the electromagnetic field equations, which led to major conceptual change in the scientific community, the effects of which continue to play out in present-day science. S2's conceptual innovation was a revision in his concept of spring to include the notion of "torsion," and though novel to himself, was already extant within science. Margaret Boden (Boden 1990) makes a useful and clarifying distinction between "P-creative" ideas that arise from episodes in which an individual creates something that is already culturally available, but novel for the individual in question, and "H-creative" ideas that arise from episodes in which something fundamentally new in human history is created. Boden focuses her attention on the nature of the mechanisms that lead to P-creative ideas, arguing, too, that examining the mundane case provides insight into the cognitive mechanisms underlying each.

While it does provide an exemplar whose subject matter is easier for nonexperts to understand than nineteenth-century physics, the P-creative reasoning in the protocol exhibits much of the complexity and power of the H-creative reasoning in the historical case. In the S2 case, we see the reasoning at work step by step. The significant parallels tend to substantiate my argument that Maxwell is likely to have gone through similar creative activity in his reasoning processes, such as mentally simulating his models and drawing while he thought. Thus, the S2 case lends support to the thesis that Maxwell used model-based reasoning, and, more generally, that conceptual change involves such reasoning.

1.5 Overview of the Book

This book synthesizes and elaborates an argument I have been developing for many years: The modeling practices of scientists found in the historical records of conceptual innovation and change constitute genuine reasoning, through which new representations are constructed. To understand the fine-structure processes of these creative achievements requires an interdisciplinary analysis that uses methods, analytical tools and concepts, and theories from philosophy, history, and cognitive science. Infusing philosophical analysis of the creative practices with research into the more "ordinary" cognitive practices can further our understanding of how they are productive forms of reasoning. The infusion, however, goes both ways—it furthers likewise a deeper understanding of cognition. Here, for instance, examining the problem-solving practices of scientists provides insights about analogy and mental modeling which show in what ways current cognitive theories could be improved.

Chapters 2 and 3 develop exemplars of successful model-based reasoning practices in conceptual change. Chapter 2 details the nature and source of the constraints that went into constructing and evaluating each of the models Maxwell built in the 1861–1862 paper, as well as in what ways analogy, imagistic, and simulative processes figure into the problem solving. By laying out the model-building processes in terms of constraints, I make evident the contributions of each domain, the target, source, and the model itself. The S2 protocol analyzed in chapter 3 was collected originally as part of an experimental investigation of expert problem solving by the cognitive scientist John Clement. The protocol is a communication of S2's heeded thought processes that emerged while solving a problem, which included developing an explanation to satisfy himself as to why the problem solution he arrived at was likely to be correct. In the process of developing that explanation, he changed his concept of spring. As noted above, the exemplar was selected because it exhibits the same kinds of reasoning through analogy, imagery, and model simulation as the Maxwell case, "writ small" but of sufficient complexity to require addressing many of the difficult issues in explaining how such reasoning practices generate new representations. Each exemplar exhibits incremental processes of model construction, manipulation, and adaptation, in which (and this turns out to be key to the process) imaginary hybrid models serve as intermediary representations between target and source domains.

The S2 exemplar offers the reader some options as to how to proceed: (1) begin with the qualitative analysis of the Maxwell case or (2) proceed directly to the second case study of the spring problem in chapter 3, through which it is still possible to come away with a sufficient understanding of the major features of the kinds of modeling practices on which I base my analysis. If the second option is taken, I highly recommend reading section 2.1, on Maxwell's problem situation, and section 2.3, which summarizes the main features and discusses in more general terms the nature of the model-based reasoning practices, since these will be referred to in subsequent chapters.

Chapter 4 proposes a cognitive basis for these practices in the human capacity for simulative thinking through mental modeling. There is as yet no consensus position that can serve as a theory of mental modeling. Thus, I first discuss foundational issues with respect to representation and reasoning, and then bring together several strands of research to develop a "minimalist" hypothesis consistent with the cognitive research and scientific practices: in certain problem-solving tasks, people reason by constructing an internal iconic model of entities, processes, situations, and events that can be manipulated by simulation. What I mean by "iconic model" is developed in the chapter. Here, as in chapter 5, I draw on and integrate research across a range of cognitive science domains.

Chapter 5 addresses the interrelationship of representation and reasoning in mental modeling. Analogies, imagistic representations, and thought experiments are cast as modes of reasoning that facilitate changing representations. I examine these as used in the exemplars, but also more broadly. In the exemplars, considerable intellectual work was required to bring together the requisite representational resources to create models through which to reason. One of my main findings is that the constructed models are imaginary hybrids of target and source domains, possessing constraints of their own as well. Not until a constructed model was established to be an adequate representation were the inferences that follow from it transferred to the target problem, which also is explicated and transformed in the process. Analogy is augmented by imagistic and simulative processes. My idea of iterative problem solving through constraint satisfaction explicates specifically what we mean when employing the metaphor of bootstrapping. Since the scientific practices are of far greater complexity than the studies developed in cognitive science, in my analysis I not only use insights from that literature, but also consider the ways in which the exemplars raise considerations beyond, and challenges to, that literature.

Chapter 6 summarizes the argument and returns to the original problem of creativity in conceptual change: given that we must start from existing representations, how can a genuinely novel representation be created? My core idea is that model-based reasoning processes facilitate and constrain the abstraction and integration of information from multiple sources and formats, enabling situations in which truly novel combinations can arise as candidate solutions to representational problems. Concepts specify constraints for generating models; conceptual innovation involves processes of creating novel sets of constraints. Through model-based reasoning, constraints abstracted from different sources can interact in ways such that a model with heretofore unrepresented structure or behaviors can emerge.

2 Model-based Reasoning Practices: Historical Exemplar

History, if viewed as a repository for more than anecdote or chronology, could produce a decisive transformation in the image of science by which we are now possessed.

—Thomas Kuhn, *The Structure of Scientific Revolutions*

In this chapter, I examine one of the most significant problem-solving episodes in the history of science, James Clerk Maxwell's first derivation of the field equations for electromagnetic phenomena. Here a fundamentally new representational structure entered physics: a quantitative field representation of forces. With this, earlier speculations about field processes in electricity and magnetism were transformed into a scientifically viable concept.

Prior to Maxwell's analysis there were two representations of forces: (1) as acting at a distance (including "potential" fields, a mathematical device for calculating action-at-a-distance forces); and (2) as transmitted continuously through a physical medium, such as water or an elastic solid. Even in the second instance, the underlying forces were assumed to be instances of Newtonian forces acting at a distance between the particles of the medium. Michael Faraday had introduced a qualitative field concept for electric and magnetic forces. He favored the interpretation that the forces are transmitted through space by means of continuous-action processes, with no underlying Newtonian medium. In contrast to Faraday's favored hypothesis, Maxwell started from the assumption that these processes are instances of the second type, transmitted through a quasi-material mechanical medium, the aether. In the problem-solving discussed here, he provided a mathematical representation for the field processes, which, if correct, would establish that electromagnetic forces are transmitted with a time delay, and thus, that the concept of field is required to describe and explain these forces.

Contrary to what Maxwell himself thought, his analysis did not incorporate the field representation of electromagnetism into the Newtonian framework as an instance of (2) above. Rather, he gave mathematical expression to a new form of representation for forces. With hindsight, we see Maxwell's problem solution as of historic significance (H-creative) because he constructed the laws of a non-Newtonian dynamical system. As we know, his work opened the door to future radical changes brought about through relativity and quantum mechanics. I have written previously about this case in a more historical vein. My interest in it in the present context is to provide an exemplar of model-based reasoning leading to conceptual change. By investigating Maxwell's modeling practices we gain significant insight into a central problem of creativity: Given that we must start from existing representations, how is it possible that genuinely novel representations are created? In the Maxwell case, the problem can be formulated as how, starting from representations of mechanical dynamical systems, did Maxwell derive the laws representing a nonmechanical dynamical system? Maxwell's electromagnetic field equations are inconsistent with Newtonian mechanics. Put another way, the field equations will not map back onto the domain from which the models through which Maxwell derived the equations were constructed.

One might construe what Maxwell did as analogical reasoning, but the practices I will discuss do not accord easily with existing accounts of analogical reasoning in philosophy or in cognitive science. There was no existing source domain solution that he could map to the electromagnetic target domain. Rather, he engaged in processes of reasoning through constructing, manipulating, evaluating, and adapting conceptual models taken to represent salient features of the phenomena under investigation. The models that he built were imaginary hybrid constructions of both domains. Analogical domains served as sources of constraints for creating and adapting models, in combination with constraints from the target domain and the models themselves. His reasoning made significant use of both mental and external representations. Finally, making sense of his reasoning, such as the question of how he came up with the source analogies, requires also that it be understood as taking place within a problem situation.

Maxwell (1861–1862) carried out the analysis in four parts. Part I concerns magnetic phenomena. Part II concerns electric currents and electromagnetic phenomena. Part III deals with static electricity. Part IV shows how the model accounts for the action of magnetism on polarized light. Parts I through III, which develop the models and derive the equations, are discussed here. My aim is first to make as compelling case as possible for the hypothesis *that* the modeling practices are generative of the representation. Then, I sketch thoughts on *how* they could have been productive, which will be elaborated after developing the second exemplar in chapter 3.

2.1 Maxwell's Problem Situation

Although our focus is on an individual's reasoning processes, as I have argued earlier, it would be mistaken to interpret the modeling practices as occurring in isolation—divorced from a social, cultural, material, and cognitive context that constitutes Maxwell's *problem situation*. To interpret his problem solving requires that we understand it as embedded in a rich fabric of community practices that provide the conceptual, analytical, and material resources employed in his research. Why did he start from a continuous-action approach to electricity and magnetism? Why did he construct analogical models? Why did he choose certain analogical source domains? These are questions that can be answered only through understanding his problem situation.

Maxwell's approach derives from the locales he inhabited, that is, where he lived, was educated, taught, and did research. The Scottish geometrical approach to using mathematics, and the related Cambridge continuum mechanical approach to physical problems, provided the contexts that shaped the nature of the theoretical, experimental, and mathematical knowledge and the methodological practices with which he formulated the problem and approached its solution. The work of Michael Faraday and William Thomson (later, Lord Kelvin) contributed most significantly to these. Continental physicists working at the same time on electromagnetism, such as Andre Ampère, employed quite different practices and drew from fundamentally different theoretical assumptions and mathematical and physical representational structures (see, e.g., Hoffman 1996). Differences in their problem situations figure into why these physicists failed to derive the field equations. Elaborating on all of the resources available in Maxwell's problem situation would make for a different book, so only a basic inventory of those resources that contributed to his construction of the field equations is provided here. More extensive discussions of some of these can be found in *Faraday to Einstein* (Nersessian 1984a) and in the various references cited below. These resources included, specifically:

1. The geometrical (physical and visual) approach to mathematics prevalent in the Scottish and Cambridge traditions (Davies 2000).

2. Faraday's experimental research, modeling practices, and theoretical interpretations (Faraday 1831–1855; Gooding 1990; Nersessian 1984a, 1985).

3. Macroscopic techniques of mathematical analysis for continuum mechanical phenomena, developed in Cambridge by Maxwell and his colleagues, specifically partial differential equations for analyzing macroscopic structure as opposed to microscopic summation of forces between particles (integration techniques) (Buchwald 1985; Siegel 1991).

4. Thomson's analysis of electrostatic lines of force in terms of partial differential equations and potential theory (Thomson 1845).

5. Thomson's "mathematical analogy" showing that the distribution of forces of linear and rotational strain in an elastic solid is analogous to the distribution of electric and magnetic forces (Thomson 1847).

6. Thomson's postulation of vortices in a medium to explain the handedness of rotation of plane of polarization (Thomson 1856).

7. Thomson's general method of analogy.

8. Work on heat, especially Thomson's (1851) "dynamical" theory of heat, where "dynamical" means forces arising from the internal motion of a system, rather than attraction and repulsion between particles. This assumes the rotational motions of individual molecules, which William Rankine called "molecular vortices," and is the source of Thomson's postulation of vortex motion for the magnetic medium in the 1856 paper (Crosbie Smith and Wise 1989; Siegel 1991).

9. The recently formulated concept of energy and its conservation.

10. The electromagnetic theories of action-at-a-distance theorists such as Ampère and Wilhelm Weber.

11. Maxwell's earlier kinematical paper on the lines of force, which provided a geometrical analysis in terms of integral equations (Maxwell 1855–1856).

12. Various machinery permeating Victorian culture, for example, the steam engine and Charles Babbage's analytical engine (Crosbie Smith and Wise 1989).

The title of Maxwell's 1861–1862 paper itself, "On physical lines of force," refers directly to Faraday's speculation about the reality of lines of force. Late in his research, Faraday distinguished between lines of force conceived purely geometrically (Faraday 1852a) and lines of force conceived as physical entities whose various motions constitute all the forces of nature (1852b). He published these papers in different venues in order to differentiate clearly between views he held as speculative (physical lines of force) and those he held established by experiment (geometrical configuration of lines of force). In his 1855–1856 paper, "On Faraday's lines of force," Maxwell provided a kinematical analysis of the geometrical configurations of the lines. In the 1861–1862 paper, his stated objective was to provide a dynamical analysis of the production of the lines, that is, of the electric and magnetic forces in the aether that give rise to the configuration of the lines. In the opening text, Maxwell referred directly to Faraday's account of magnetism in terms of lines of force representing the intensity and direction of the force at a point in space. His account provided Maxwell with several visual and simulative models of electric and magnetic actions.

Faraday had attempted to articulate, both experimentally and theoretically, the speculation of Oersted and others that physical processes in the regions surrounding bodies and charges might contribute to their actions upon one another. Constructing and reasoning from visual models figures prominently in Faraday's practices. Faraday had hypothesized that the lines of force that form when iron filings are sprinkled around magnets and charged matter indicate that a real physical process is going on in the space surrounding these objects and that this process is part of the transmission of the actions (Faraday 1831–1855). The visual display made by iron filings, for example, as they take on a geometrical configuration around a magnetic source, had a profound influence on the understanding of electric and magnetic actions, and of forces and matter in general, that Faraday developed. Figure 2.1 shows a plate of actual configurations of lines of force. Figure 2.2 shows Faraday's schematic rendering of the lines around a bar magnet.

I have argued in earlier work (Nersessian 1984a, 1985) that as Faraday's theory developed, this image came to represent not only the geometrical shape of the lines, but also a dynamical model of their actions. The model is dynamical in that although the visual representation on paper is of a static geometrical pattern, Faraday reasoned with it as representing dynamic processes (see also Gooding 1980, 1990; Tweney 1992). For instance, he envisioned the various forces of nature as motions in the lines, such as waving, bending, stretching, and vibrating. On his full conceptualization of force, all the forces of nature are unified and interconvertible through various motions of the lines of force, with matter as point-centers of converging lines of force.

Near the end of his research, Faraday introduced another visual model that was to play a key role in Maxwell's work. He represented the interconvertibility of electricity and magnetism through motion by means of a

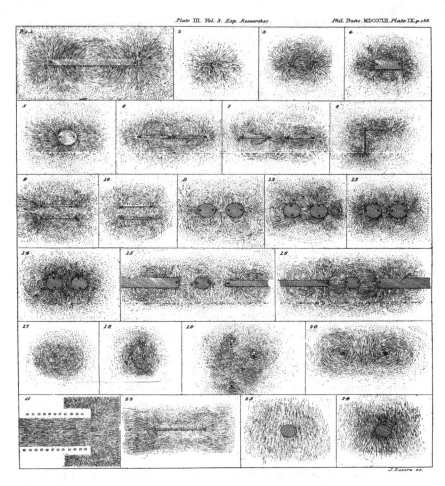

Figure 2.1
Actual patterns of lines of force around various sources. Faraday 1831–1852, volume 3, plate III.

diagram of curves interlocking at right angles to one another, as shown in figure 2.3.

This visual model represents the dynamic balance between electricity and magnetism; the "oneness of condition of that which is apparently two powers or forms of power" (Faraday 1831–1855, 3, para. 3268). That is, as one ring expands or contracts, the other makes a reciprocal motion.

The model is an abstraction from two previous models, both also represented visually. First, as represented in figure 2.4, on the lines of force model, the balance lies in the notion that magnetic lines repel laterally,

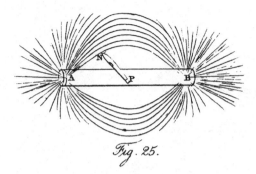

Figure 2.2
Faraday's drawing of lines of force. Faraday 1831–1852, volume 1, plate I, series 1, figure 25.

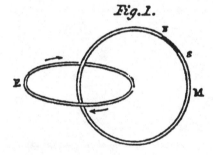

Figure 2.3
Faraday's interlocking rings; Faraday 1831–1852, volume 3, plate IV, figure 1.

which has the same effect as a longitudinal expansion of electric current lines, and contract longitudinally, which has the same effect as a lateral attraction of electric current lines. Second, it derives from an intermediate sketch made a few months after his discovery of electromagnetic induction, shown in figure 2.5, which Faraday drew in his diary while trying to understand the dynamical relations among electricity, magnetism, and motion.

The balance here lies in their interactions. In the discussion where it appears, Faraday comments that it is to be understood as a dynamic representation that admits of many combinations, in which any of the lines can be taken to represent electricity, magnetism, or motion.

Maxwell's first paper on electricity and magnetism (1855–1856) provided a mathematical formulation for Faraday's notions of "quantity" (magnetic

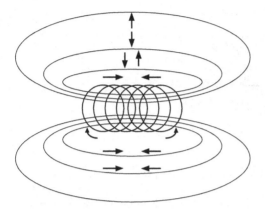

Figure 2.4
My schematic representation of the reciprocal relationship between magnetic lines
of force and electric current lines.

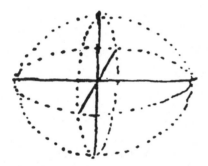

Figure 2.5
Faraday's unified representation of electricity, magnetism, and motion; *Diary* entry,
March 26, 1832.

force summed across the lines, and so related to the density of lines in a
region) and "intensity" (magnetic force related to the tension along the
lines) as "flux" and "flow" respectively. He replaced Faraday's discrete
measure of intensity in terms of "number of" lines cut with a continuous
function. Faraday's model of dynamical balance, embodied in figure 2.3,
which Maxwell called *"mutually embracing* curves" (Maxwell 1890a, 1:194n),
is reflected in Maxwell's mathematical representations for the field. He
used two fields each—one for "intensity" (force) and one for "quantity"
(flux)—for the electric and magnetic forces, giving eight equations instead
of the four that are now customary. Norton Wise (1979) has provided a

convincing account of the role of this visual model in Maxwell's analysis. Wise also suggested that mentally simulating the image could have provided Maxwell with a model of propagation of electromagnetic actions. If one imagines expanding the two interlocked rings in figure 2.3 into a linked chain, this has the effect of propagating the summaries of the quantities and intensities associated with the electric and magnetic fields link by link. In this way, "the mutual embrace now became productive of offspring" (Wise 1979, 1316). It is important to note, though, that on Maxwell's analysis propagation of the force is neither along nor through the lines of force, but orthogonal to them.

In setting up the 1861–1862 analysis Maxwell imagined an experiment that relates his motivations directly to Faraday's notion of the *physical* lines of force: "if we strew iron filings on paper near a magnet each filing would be magnetized by induction and the consecutive filings will unite by their opposite poles, so as to form fibers, and those fibers will *indicate* the direction of the lines of force. The beautiful illustration of the presence of magnetic force afforded by this experiment, naturally tends to make us think of the lines of force as something real" (451, emphasis in the original). Maxwell also referred to the paper of his friend and teacher Thomson (Thomson 1847) in which Thomson had constructed analogies between the aether and elastic media under stress, for the purpose of representing the magnitude and direction of electric, magnetic, and current forces in a medium. Thomson's analysis was purely geometrical. Maxwell had already followed Thomson in using analogical models to solve representational problems in his 1855–1856 paper. In an extensive correspondence with Thomson while he was working on these papers, Maxwell acknowledged his debt to him for what he called the method of "physical analogy" and even went so far as to express the belief that Thomson might have anticipated some of his results (Larmor 1937, 17–18). Physical analogy, according to Maxwell, is a "method of investigation, which allows the mind at every step to lay hold of a clear physical conception, without being committed to any theory founded on the physical science from which that conception is borrowed" (Maxwell 1855–1856, 156). A "physical analogy" is "that partial similarity between the laws of one science and those of another which makes each of them illustrate the other" (ibid.).

As Howard Stein has pointed out, " 'analogy' in Maxwell's sense is an isomorphism, an equivalence of form" (Stein 1976, 35). This much can be said, however, of the many analogies Thomson constructed, such as between heat and electrostatics: There is an important difference with respect to physical analogies that is critical to understanding how Maxwell

was able to create a fundamentally novel representation. As Maxwell wrote
to Thomson, "I intend to borrow it for a season . . . but applying it in a
somewhat different way" (Larmor 1937, May 15, 1855, p. 11; see also letters
of November 13, 1854; May 18, 1855, 8, 11; and September 13, 1855, 17–
18.) The difference is that Maxwell used what might be considered analogical source domains not as providing for direct mappings between
phenomena, but as sources for constraints. These constraints were incorporated into imaginary models that are *hybrid representations* of the source
domain and target phenomena. The model then becomes an analogical
source itself and isomorphic mappings are made between the models on
their mechanical interpretation and the models on their electromagnetic
interpretation. I discuss these differences further after developing the specifics of Maxwell's modeling processes.

Maxwell's model-based reasoning practices involved constructing, evaluating, and adapting models through processes of abstracting and integrating various constraints. The constraints are empirical, mathematical, and
theoretical in nature. They derive from a variety of sources: from the
domains of continuum mechanics and machine mechanics, from experimental findings in electricity and magnetism, and from mathematics, as
well as from various hypotheses of Faraday and Thomson. Once Maxwell
formulated a satisfactory model representing a specific mechanism, he
considered those abstract relational structures of the mechanical model
that could account for the electromagnetic phenomena, formulated the
equations of the abstract model, and substituted in the electromagnetic
variables. Each model presented in the paper works for solving a piece of
the problem. Each model builds on the previous model—though not in a
totally coherent manner. Unlike the S2 protocol exemplar developed in
the next chapter, there is no record of possible discarded models. It is
unclear just how much drafting Maxwell ever committed to paper, as a fire
destroyed most of his records. Only fragments of calculations—indicating
some alternative considerations—remain and are now published in his
Collected Papers (Harman 1990, 1995).

In presenting this case I will not specify all the constraints used in constructing the three models, providing instead a streamlined version that
focuses on those most significant for understanding the model-construc-
tive processes. Contrary to our current understanding of them, current and
charges are taken to be the *result* of stresses in the medium and not the
sources of fields. This is reflected in the form of Maxwell's equations, where
the field quantities appear to the right of the equal sign, rather than to the
left as is the current custom.

2.2 Maxwell's Modeling Processes

In this and the S2 case in chapter 3, I analyze the modeling processes in such a way as to highlight the various constraints involved in construction, manipulation, and adaptation. In doing so, my intent is to make evident the contributions of target, source, and model to these reasoning processes. In these exemplars, novel representational structures arise through the integration of the various constraints.

2.2.1 Model 1: Vortex Fluid

Maxwell's initial constraints (I) derive from his background goals and assumptions, and are intimately connected to resources in the problem situation outlined above, especially his understanding of it as encompassing experiments, theories, and mathematical results of Faraday and Thomson. He began by referring to Faraday's account of magnetism for which his 1855–1856 paper had provided a kinematical analysis of the geometrical relations among the lines of force. By contrast, the purpose of his 1861–1862 paper was to provide a dynamical analysis of the underlying mechanisms by which the tensions and motions in a medium (electromagnetic aether) could produce the observed phenomena. He expressed the hope that this investigation would lead to a unified theory of the production, transmission, and interaction of electricity, magnetism, and current, as taking place in an electromagnetic medium. As support he referred to Thomson's 1847 paper which construed the aether as an elastic medium under stress for the purposes of representing the magnitude and direction of electric, magnetic, and current forces in a medium. Based on this discussion, the initial, global, constraints (I) on the solution included:

I1. The mathematical representation should provide a unified account of the production and transmission of electric and magnetic forces.
I2. The forces are transmitted continuously in a mechanical medium, namely, the aether.

Given these constraints in Maxwell's problem situation, continuum mechanics is the obvious source domain (S) on which to model the electromagnetic aether. Continuous-action phenomena, such as fluid flow, heat, and elasticity, had all recently been given mathematical formulations in dynamical analyses consistent with Newtonian mechanics. This work was carried out primarily at Cambridge, and Maxwell had made significant contributions to it. The presumption of these analyses was that microlevel action-at-a-distance forces in the medium are responsible for macrolevel phenomena. Continuum-mechanical analyses are carried out at the macrolevel, with transmission of force treated as continuous. The initial constraints lead to the assumption that dynamical relations that hold in pertinent areas of continuum mechanics will also hold in electromagnetism.

The target constraints (T) are those specific to electricity and magnetism. The initial target constraints Maxwell mentions were derived from Faraday's experiments and his and Thomson's interpretations of them:

T1. There is a tension along the lines of force.
T2. There is a lateral repulsion between the lines of force.
T3. The electric and magnetic actions are at right angles to one another.
T4. A plane of polarized light is rotated by the action of magnetism.

Maxwell began with discussing general features of stress in a medium. Stress results from action and reaction of the contiguous parts of a medium and "consists in general of pressure or tensions different in different directions at the same point in the medium" (1861–1862, 454). On the initial constraint, I2, one can assume that the causes of electromagnetic phenomena are stresses in the aether and thus assume that there is a "resemblance in form" between dynamical relations that hold in the domains of continuum mechanics, such as fluids and elastic solids, and electromagnetic phenomena. In considering the nature of the stresses in a continuum-mechanical medium that could accommodate the target constraints, Maxwell inferred as possible source constraints:

S1. There is a tension in the direction of the lines of force.
S2. Pressure is greater in the equatorial than in the axial direction.

The source constraint S1 satisfies target constraint T1 because in both attraction and repulsion an object is drawn in the direction of the resultant of the lines of force. S2 satisfies T2 because an object would experience a lateral repulsion, as occurs between the lines of force.

Maxwell determined that a fluid medium with a hydrostatic pressure symmetrical around the axis and a simple pressure along the axis provides a mechanical model consistent with the two source constraints. The excess pressure in the equatorial direction can be explained as the result of the centrifugal force of vortices in the medium, with axes parallel to the lines of force. That is, the medium would have rotational motion, with the direction of rotation determined by T3 so as to produce lines of force in the same direction (what physicists now call "handedness") as those about a current.

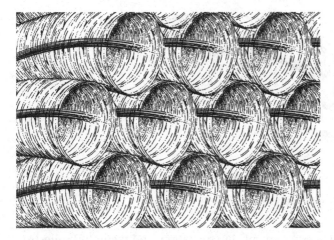

Figure 2.6
My rendering of the vortex medium from Maxwell's description.

Although Maxwell did not refer directly to Thomson's 1856 paper in which he proposed that vortex motion in the medium could account for the rotation of a plane of polarized light passed through a magnetic field, the title of Part I of Maxwell's paper, "The theory of molecular vortices applied to magnetic phenomena," makes implicit reference to it. The vortex fluid model satisfies all the target constraints thus far, plus an implicit empirical constraint:

T5. Magnetism is dipolar.

That is, taking figure 2.7 to represent a single vortex, if one looks from the south pole (small end) toward the north pole of the magnet along a line of force, the vortex moves clockwise. Maxwell needed only to consider such a single vortex in his analysis of various magnetic phenomena.

The system of infinitesimal vortices, however, does not correspond to any known physical system, and is thus does not provide a ready-to-hand analogue. The vortex fluid model incorporates constraints from both domains, and so it represents *both* hydrodynamics and magnetism in the salient respects. In reasoning with it, one needs to understand the model as satisfying constraints that apply to possible *types* of entities and processes that can be considered as constituting either domain. Reasoning through the model enabled Maxwell to draw on the mathematical representational structures of continuum mechanics to derive the equations for

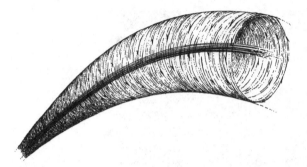

Figure 2.7
My rendering of a single vortex from Maxwell's description.

the stresses on the hydrodynamic interpretation, and then on the electromagnetic interpretation. The procedure he used throughout was: (1) construct a model; (2) derive a mathematical representation on the continuum mechanical interpretation; (3) construct a mapping between the quantities and relations of the model and the electromagnetic quantities and relations to rewrite the equations for the latter; and (4) evaluate the electromagnetic interpretation.

The vortex model captures significant implicit geometric and quantitative constraints matching a rich set of constraints that hold of Faraday's lines of force, as Maxwell had analyzed them in the earlier, kinematical paper. He does not make these explicit here, but for having said at the outset that his objective was to give a dynamical explanation of the lines. Examples of geometrical constraints are those relating to the configuration of the experimentally produced magnetic lines of force, such as lines between two magnets whose attracting poles are near each other or connecting the poles of a single magnet (see figure 2.1). The configuration constraints are satisfied by the shape of each vortex. The reader should look at figure 2.7 while following along with my descriptions here. A vortex is wider the farther it is from its origin, which gives the system the property that lines become farther apart as they approach their midpoints.

Examples of quantitative constraints are those relating to magnetic intensity, such as that a point on a less central line of force between two magnets has a lower magnetic intensity or that the magnetic intensity increases for a point moving along a line of force from its midpoint to its end. The variation of intensity along a line of force corresponds to a decrease in the circumferential velocity of a vortex as one moves from its origin. The variation of intensity as one moves away from the axis

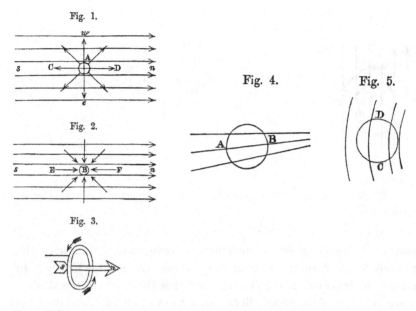

Figure 2.8
Maxwell's cross-sectional drawings of vortices and lines of force. Maxwell 1890a, volume 1, 460.

corresponds to the greater width of vortices that are farther from the axis, and thus have less velocity at corresponding points. Variables pertaining to the strength of a magnet and permeability correspond to pressure along the axis and density of vortices in the medium, respectively, with a stronger magnet corresponding to greater pressure, and lower density corresponding to greater permeability. These quantitative properties of fluid media satisfy the constraints on the velocity around a vortex, which are needed for continuum mechanics to serve as a source domain from which to construct a model. The vortex motion supplies a causal mechanism that is in principle capable of producing the configuration of the lines of force and the stresses in and among them.

Maxwell's most significant derivation from this model was the "stress tensor," which represents the resultant force on an element of the magnetic medium due to its internal stress. In discussing the interpretation of the mathematical result, he provided visual representations of the configuration of the vortices and the lines of force for north and south magnetic poles (see figure 2.8), accompanied by text instructing the reader how to imagine the motion of the vortices in the planes above and below the

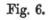

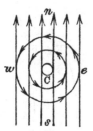

Figure 2.9
Maxwell's drawing of a cross section of lines of force around a wire. Maxwell 1890a,
volume 1, 463.

plane of the paper on which the figures are drawn and how to relate the
motions to mechanical effects of the vortices. We are, for instance, to
imagine in Maxwell's figures 1 through 3 that the "parts of the vortices
above the plane of the paper will be moving towards e [east], and the parts
below that plane towards w [west]" (459).

Two further derivations make explicit significant target constraints not
discussed by Maxwell before in the analysis. Any adequate model would
need to satisfy Ampère's law relating current and magnetism and, in the
limit, the action-at-a-distance inverse square law, Coulomb's law, as Faraday
had generalized it for media of varying density. Using the electromagnetic
substitution mapping constructed for the stress tensor, Maxwell derived a
mathematical expression relating current density to the circulation of the
magnetic field around the current-carrying wire that satisfied Ampère's law
in the differential form he had derived in the 1855–1856 paper (Maxwell
1890a, 1:194). This new derivation was not based on a model representation of a causal mechanism connecting current and magnetism; it is
descriptive just as in the earlier paper. Maxwell accompanied the derivation with an illustration (figure 2.9) of the motion of the vortices and
configuration of the resulting lines of force around a wire. He also provided
a description for how to imagine the motion.

This derivation established that in the limiting case of no currents in the
medium and a unified magnetic permeability, the inverse square law of
Coulomb could be derived. Maxwell also derived differential forms of the
law for more general cases, involving currents and various media such as
air and water. Thus the model satisfied the implicit target constraint that
it be consistent under the appropriate conditions with established mathematical results:

T6. The model agrees with Ampère's law.

T7. The model agrees in the limit with Coulomb's law.

In the analysis up to this point, Maxwell had been able to use mathematical properties of individual vortices to derive a mathematical representation for magnetic induction, paramagnetism, and diamagnetism consistent with the known constraints on magnetic systems. The vortex-fluid model constructed in Part I was the starting point for the remainder of Maxwell's analysis. All subsequent reasoning was based on modifications of it.

Thus far we have considered how the source and target domains placed constraints on the model. In the next section we will see how manipulating the model itself generated constraints (M) that figured in further construction of his models.

2.2.2 Model 2: Vortex–Idle Wheel

Maxwell began Part II of the analysis by stating that its purpose was to inquire into the connection between the magnetic vortices and current, which is necessary to satisfy the initial constraint I1. The adaptation of the vortex-fluid model in this part of the analysis derived from a constraint arising from the model. Analyzing the dynamical relationships between current and magnetism required altering Model 1 to provide a mechanism connecting them. The model itself gives rise to the question of how the vortices are set in motion, and addressing this issue should lead to a representation of the relations between electricity and magnetism. Maxwell's calculations thus far had ignored interactions between adjacent vortices, focusing the analysis of the magnetic phenomena on a single vortex. Technically this is justified by assuming negligible forces between the vortices. However, a dynamical explanation of electromagnetism could not ignore these forces. Maxwell began the analysis by admitting there was a serious problem with the model: "I have found great difficulty in conceiving of the existence of vortices in a medium, side by side, revolving in the same direction" (1861–1862, 468). Figure 2.10, which is my rendering of a cross section from Maxwell's descriptions and diagrams, makes the problem evident.

On imagining the vortices in motion, we see that direct contact between the vortices will create friction, and thus jamming. Additionally, since all the vortices are rotating in the same direction and, thus, at points of contact they are going in opposite directions, in the case where they are revolving at the same rate, the whole mechanism should eventually stop. Thus, the model furnishes the constraint:

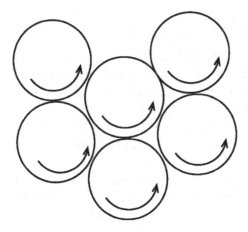

Figure 2.10
My drawing of a cross section of the vortex model.

M1. Friction is produced where the vortices come into contact.

An adapted model would have to accommodate this constraint by creating a way of separating the vortices, yet keeping them in motion. Maxwell stated that "[t]he only conception that has aided me in conceiving of this kind of motion is that of the vortices being separated by a layer of particles, acting as idle wheels is interposed between each vortex and the next, so that each vortex has a tendency to make the neighbouring vortices revolve in the same direction as itself" (ibid., 468). He noted that in the design of machinery that requires rotating parts to move smoothly past each other this kind of problem is solved by the introduction of "idle wheels." He proposed to adapt the model in a similar manner.

However, ordinary idle wheels encountered in machines rotate in place, and thus could only represent the case of an insulator. To represent the motion of a current in the conductor, the idle wheel particles needed to be capable of translational motion. Maxwell noted that there are idle wheels of this kind in the source domain of machine mechanics, such as "in epicyclic trains and other contrivances, as, for instance, Siemens's governor for steam-engines" (ibid., 469). He then went on to show that if the translational motion of the particles were taken to represent the flow of electric current, the expected distribution of lines of force would occur. He introduced an analogy and diagram (figure 2.11) with another kind of mechanical gear configuration, a "toothed wheel or a rack to wheels which it drives" (ibid., 472), which exemplifies "the line of magnetic force

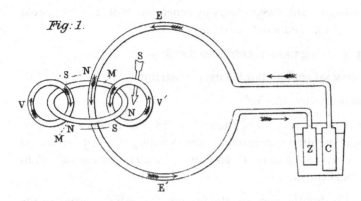

Figure 2.11
Maxwell's drawing of a mechanism through which motion of the particles between vortices V and V' would create magnetic lines of force MM'; Maxwell 1890a, volume 1, plate VIII, figure 1.

embracing the electric circuit" (ibid.) that relates directly to the Faraday diagram (figure 2.3) discussed earlier.

In this analysis of how the motion of the particles could represent current, Maxwell is not making use of any existing mechanism; rather he is working with a class of mechanisms of a specific *type*. His analysis worked directly with the imagined modification of the original model to determine specific features of the modification—generic idle wheel particles—based on constraints of electromagnetic phenomena and of the model. For example, specific idealizations about the relations among the particles— that there is no slipping and that they do not touch when rotating in place—are dictated by the additional target constraint:

T8. The lines of force surrounding a constant magnetic source can exist for an indefinite time.

This, in turn, became salient in working out the nature of the model mechanism. For the model, T8 corresponds to the constraint on the mechanism:

M2. There is no loss of energy when the particles are rotating in place.

In translational motion, however, which represents the case of a current, the particles would experience resistance so that energy is lost and heat created. That is, for the particles to be in translational motion, the vortices would need to have differing velocities. As the particles moved, they would experience resistance and waste energy by generating heat, as is consistent with currents. Thus, the model constraint

M3. Resistance during motion creates energy loss

satisfies the now salient additional target constraint

T9. Heat loss occurs by currents.

Finally, as with the analysis of the first model, this model also had to satisfy various quantitative constraints. For example, Maxwell considered the angular velocity as constant to simplify calculations, which yielded an additional model constraint:

M4. There is no slipping between the interior and exterior layers of the vortices.

In the mathematical analysis of Part II, this constraint required treating the vortices as rigid pseudospheres. So conceived, the vortices now appear to be inconsistent with the implicit geometrical constraints of the vortices in Part I, which on the face of it require them to be elastic. Maxwell did not address this problem here, but it would turn out to be key in the modification of the model in his analysis of electrostatics in Part III.

The resulting vortex–idle wheel model is a hybrid construction, with two source domains, fluid dynamics and machine mechanics, satisfying constraints from these, electromagnetism, and features of the model itself. Throughout this section—as in the rest of Part II—Maxwell derived the equations for the relations between particles and vortices in the model and then constructed mappings between the model and target electromagnetic phenomena. He noted where the new results were consistent with those derived earlier. One significant result was that the flux density of the particles was shown to represent the electric current density, satisfying T6.

In discussing results, he provided analogies with plausible machine mechanisms, as exemplars of specific relations he derived between the idle wheel particles and the fluid vortices to establish that there are real physical systems that instantiate the generic relations of the model. Figure 2.12 is most interesting in that it again explicitly references the interlocking rings of figure 2.3 by Faraday, once more using the language of *"embrace,"* where C is a conducting wire embracing the induction ring B. Maxwell used this drawing to illustrate what he called an *"experiment"* (ibid., 478) which he carried out in thought.

The point of the experiment was to determine if the model captured known phenomena of electromagnetic induction. Essentially, altering the

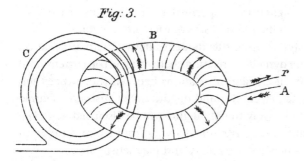

Figure 2.12
Maxwell's representation of a thought experiment of how an electromotive force induces a current on the model. Maxwell 1890a, volume 1, plate VIII, figure 3.

velocity of the vortices through the action of the idle wheel particles should induce a current.

Once he had established that indeed the relations between currents and magnetism could be represented by the vortex–idle wheel model, Maxwell then proceeded to consider the dynamical forces in the model that could give rise to known electrodynamical phenomena. Before moving on to an outline of that analysis, it is important to heed Maxwell's explanation of how he is reasoning with the model, and how the inferences he makes should be understood. He stressed that the idle wheel mechanism was not to be considered "a mode of connexion existing in nature" (ibid., 486). Rather, it is "a mode of connexion which is mechanically conceivable and easily investigated, and it serves to bring out the actual mechanical connexions between the known electro-magnetic phenomena" (ibid.). In reality, the idle wheel mechanism is a highly implausible mode of connection for a fluid mechanical system. What Maxwell is pointing out here is that, even so, the *relational structures* among the forces producing stresses in the model do correspond to the *relational structures* among forces between current electricity and magnetism. Maxwell's hypothesis is that they belong to the same class of mechanical systems, not that they are the same mechanical phenomena. The "pressure on the axle of a wheel" (ibid.) under conditions specific to the purposes of the problem at hand, for example, is a phenomenon belonging to a class of mechanical systems that are capable of producing the kinds of stresses associated with the electromotive force in a mechanical electromagnetic aether; but it is not the same phenomenon. What is driving the analysis is the assumption that the *dynamical relations* between the idle wheels and vortices are of the *same kind* as those between current and magnetism as specified within the context of this problem, not that the specific mechanisms of each are the same.

Maxwell was successful in using this model to derive the mathematical equations governing the dynamical relations between electric currents and magnetism in terms of the dynamical relations between the vortices and the idle wheels. Many target, model, and quantitative constraints figured into this analysis, of which only the highlights will be discussed here. The most salient additional target constraints deriving from empirical investigations of the relations between electricity and magnetism are:

T10. A steady current produces magnetic lines of force around it.
T11. Starting or stopping a current produces a current, with opposite orientation, in a conducting wire parallel to it.
T12. Motion of a conductor across the magnetic lines of force induces a current in it.

We can see how the model satisfies constraints T10 through 12, by referring to Maxwell's representation of the model conceived as in motion.

Note that to exhibit packing, Maxwell used hexagons in a cross-sectional view of dodecahedra, which approximate spheres in the limit (figure 2.13). The diagrammatic representation of the model is accompanied by text to animate it correctly:

Let the current from left to right commence in AB. the row of vortices gh above AB will be set in motion in the opposite direction to a watch. . . . We shall suppose the row of vortices kl still at rest, then the layer of particles between these rows will be acted on by the row gh on their lower sides and will be at rest above. If they are free to move, they will rotate in the negative direction, and will at the same time move from right to left, or in the opposite direction from the current, and so form an *induced* electric current. (Maxwell 1890a, vol. 1, 477, emphasis in the original)

He continued in this vein with instructions for how to see other induction phenomena through animating the diagram until concluding: "[I]t appears therefore that the phenomena of induced currents are part of the process of communicating the rotary velocity of the vortices from one part of the field to another" (ibid.).

As one illustration, we can see how the causal relationship between a steady current and magnetic lines of force is captured in the following way. A continuous flow of particles is needed to maintain the configuration of the magnetic lines of force about a current. When an electromotive force, such as from a battery, acts on the particles in a conductor, it pushes them and starts them rolling. The tangential pressure between them and the vortices sets the neighboring vortices in motion in opposite directions on

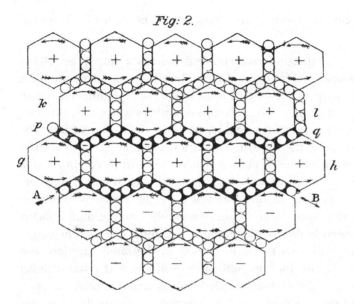

Figure 2.13
Maxwell's representation of electromagnetic induction through the vortex–idle wheel mechanism. Maxwell 1890a, volume 1, plate VIII, figure 2.

opposite sides—thus capturing the polarity of magnetism (T5)—and this motion is transmitted throughout the medium. The mathematical expression Maxwell derived connects current with the rotating torque the vortices exert on the particles. The translational velocity of the particles is half the difference between the velocities of the vortices on either side of it, which satisfies T10. Maxwell showed this equation to be consistent with the equations he had derived in Part I for the distribution and configuration of the magnetic lines of force around a steady current.

Another way the model is driving Maxwell's reasoning is that the mechanics of this model differ for the two primary cases of electromagnetic induction, and so the derivation was carried out in two parts. Given the target constraints (T11 and T12) there is no reason to view the two cases of electromagnetic induction asymmetrically; but on the model, the cases have different causes. The first case concerns an electromotive force on a stationary conductor produced by a changing magnetic field. This case corresponds to T11, the constraint that induction occurs, for example, when a current is switched off and on in a conducting loop, and produces a current in the reverse direction in a nearby conducting loop. This constraint can be restated as

T11′. A changing (nonhomogeneous) magnetic field induces a current in a conductor.

On the model, a changing magnetic field induces a current as follows (the reader should look at figure 2.13 while reading my description). A decrease or increase in the current will cause a corresponding change in velocity in the adjacent vortices. The row of vortices where the conductor is located will have a different velocity from the next adjacent row. The difference will cause the idle-wheel particles surrounding those vortices to speed up or slow down, a motion that will in turn be communicated to the next row of vortices, and so on until the second conducting wire is reached. The particles in that wire will be set in translational motion by the differential electromotive force between the vortices, thus inducing a current oriented in direction opposite to the initial current. The neighboring vortices will then be set in motion in the same direction, and the resistance in the medium ultimately will cause the translational motion to stop, so that the particles will then only rotate in place and there will be no induced current. Figure 2.12 specifically illustrates this mechanism.

The second case is that satisfying constraint T12, where a current is induced by motion of a conductor across the lines of force. When a conducting wire moves across the medium, it creates a deformation of the vortices and thus a change in velocity. Maxwell used considerations about the changing form and position of the fluid medium in the analysis. Briefly (again, the reader should look at figure 2.13 while reading my description), the portion of the medium in the direction of the motion of a conducting wire becomes compressed by the wire, causing the vortices to elongate and speed up. Behind the wire the vortices will contract back into place and decrease in velocity. The net force will push the idle-wheel particles inside the conductor, producing a current provided there is a circuit connecting the ends of the wire.

After he derived the mathematical representation for each induction mechanism, Maxwell provided an extensive set of instructions for how to visualize the relationships among the lines, the vortices, and the conductor (1861–1862, 483–485) and provided two diagrams, figures 4 and 5, plate VIII (figure 2.14).

We are told, for instance, to view the wire as perpendicular to the axes of the vortices and moving east to west across a system of lines of force running north to south; thus the particles will be running through the wire in the direction that is perpendicular to (i.e., coming out of the plane

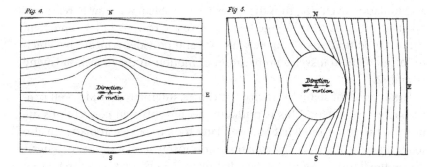

Figure 2.14
Maxwell's drawings of the lines of force surrounding, respectively, a stationary conductor (figure 4) and a moving conductor (figure 5). Maxwell 1890a, volume 1, plate VIII.

of) the paper, in which case the electromotive force is "positive when the vortices then move the interjacent particles *upwards* perpendicularly to the plane of the paper" (ibid., 484, emphasis in the original). His description of the figures tells the reader how to understand the electromagnetic phenomena in terms of the vortex–idle wheel model.

At the end of this section of his analysis, Maxwell had given mathematical expression to significant electromagnetic phenomena in terms of forces in a mechanical medium and had shown that the model satisfies salient constraints deriving from known target phenomena. The analysis thus far did not fully satisfy the initial constraints I1 and I2. For this he still needed to: (1) establish that continuous action in a medium is essential for the transmission of electromagnetic forces, that is, show that there is a necessary time delay in the propagation of the action and calculate the velocity of the propagation in the medium; and (2) incorporate static electricity into the model.

Representing static electricity required making additional adaptations to the model, which provided the means for calculating the time delay in transmission of the action. That Part III of the paper was published eight months after Parts I and II indicates that Maxwell did not see how to make the modification at the initial time of publication of the first two parts. In one sense this is surprising. Given the correspondence between the flux density of the idle wheel particles and electric current, a natural extension of the model would have been to identify excess accumulation of the particles with charge. However, the equations Maxwell had derived from the model were applicable only to closed circuits, which do not allow accumulation of charge; thus the unresolved problem was how to represent open circuits. Adapting the model to resolve the representational problem led to a modification of Ampère's law, T6, and provided a means by which to calculate the transverse propagation of motion in the model, satisfying I1 and I2.

The analysis of static electricity has caused interpreters of Maxwell considerable puzzlement. This is primarily because his sign conventions are not what is now—and what Maxwell later took to be—customary. He also made an error in sign in the equation for transmission of transverse effects in the medium. These issues have led many commentators to argue that the models played little or no role in Maxwell's analysis, with one going so far as to charge Maxwell with falsifying his results and cooking up the model after he had derived the equations by formal means (Duhem 1914). I have argued that understanding Maxwell as reasoning with Model 3 and as drawing on previous work on elasticity provides the basis for all the so-called errors except one, which can easily be interpreted as a substitution error (Nersessian 1984a,b). Additional support for my contention, however, comes from considering the question of why might Maxwell have taken so long to arrive at what seems a relatively simple modification of the model—that the vortices have elasticity. Daniel Siegel (1991), in his detailed historical analysis of the vortex–idle wheel model, has made a convincing argument that Maxwell could not immediately work out the case for open currents because in Model 2 a discontinuity would occur at the interface between the vortex–idle wheel mechanism and a dielectric substance. This discontinuity leads to an inconsistency between the Ampère law (as formulated in T6) and an additional target constraint that becomes salient in considering open circuits:

T13. There is continuity of charge.

Siegel's interpretation strengthens my case for the productive role of the models in Maxwell's thinking. The delay occurred because Maxwell needed to figure a way to adapt Model 2 so as to make the two constraints consistent.[1]

2.2.3 Model 3: Elastic Vortex–Idle Wheel
As with Model 2, the adaptation leading to Model 3 arose from a constraint on the model as a mechanical system. In Model 2, the cells of rotating fluid are separated by particles that are very small in comparison to them. When Maxwell considered the transmission of rotation from one vortex cell to another via the tangential action between the surface

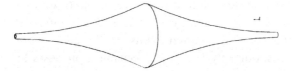

Figure 2.15
Pseudosphere.

of the vortices and the particles, he had assumed the vortices to approximate rigid pseudospheres on rotation, to simplify calculations (figure 2.15).

Now he acknowledged, however, that a salient constraint of all versions of the model as a mechanical system is:

M5. Rotation is transmitted from the exterior to the interior parts of the vortices.

To satisfy this constraint he endowed the vortex cell material with elasticity. Note that if the molecular vortices are spherical blobs of elastic material, they would also have the right configuration on rotation to satisfy the geometrical constraints discussed in section 2.3.1. That is, they would be "toplike" elastic blobs on rotation (see figures 2.7 and 2.15).

Explicitly recognizing the elastic nature of the vortices provided the means for representing static charge on the model. Maxwell began that analysis by noting the constraint:

T14. "Electric tension" associated with a charged body is the same, experimentally, whether produced from static or current electricity.

A difference in tension in a body will produce either current or static charge, depending on whether it is a conductor or insulator. Maxwell stated that in the process of electrostatic induction, electricity can be viewed as "displaced" within a molecule of a dielectric, so that one side becomes positive and the other negative, but does not pass from molecule to molecule. He then stated that although this displacement is not a current, change in displacement is "the commencement of a current" (1861–1862, 491). So, looking at the representation in figure 2.13 and imagining the vortices as elastic (Model 3), we see that during electrostatic induction, the electrostatic force produces a slight elastic distortion in the vortices, causing a slight translational motion in the idle wheel particles, which is propagated throughout the medium. This motion is what became known as the "displacement current."

It is important to understand that without the model, there is no basis on which to talk about a "current" at all. It is the translational motion of the idle wheel particles that constitutes current. Thus the derivation of the "displacement current" arises directly from the mechanical processes in the model. Recall the difference Maxwell specified between conductors and dielectrics when he first introduced the idle wheel particles. In a conductor, they are free to move from vortex to vortex. In a dielectric, they can only rotate in place. During electrostatic induction (dielectric media), the particles are urged forward by the elastic distortion of the vortices in response to the force, but since they are constrained to rotate in place in the dielectric medium, the particles react back on the vortices with a force to restore their position. This mechanism is represented in the equation that relates the electromotive force and the displacement by the orientation of the displacement in the direction opposite from what is customary now and in Maxwell's later work. The difference in sign can, thus, be accounted for by recognizing that an elastic restoring force *for the model* is opposite in orientation to the impressed force, and so the two quantities *should* have opposing signs. Without the model, there is no clear way of accounting for the sign difference.

The motion of the particles in this process is similar to the "commencement of a current" (actually, a reverse current), since their forward movement causes a brief propagation of displacement in the medium. However, the motion "does not amount to a current, because when it has attained a certain value it remains constant" (ibid., 491). That is, the system reaches a certain level of stress and remains there. Charge, then, can be represented as the excess of tension in the dielectric medium created by the accumulation of displaced idle wheel particles. This is consistent with both Faraday's and Maxwell's conception of the field as giving rise to charge (and currents), unlike the contemporary understanding of fields as arising from charges (and currents). In sum, without the model, "displacement current" does not have a physical meaning, which is what bothered so many readers of the *Treatise*, (Maxwell 1891) where the mechanical model is no longer used. Its connection to Model 3 also created difficulties for Maxwell's 1864 analysis (Nersessian 2002a).

After some further derivations that I will pass over, Maxwell addressed the need to modify the equation for Ampère's law to include "the effect due to elasticity in the medium" (1861–1862, 496). That is, since the vortices are elastic, and since in a conductor the particles are free to move, the current produced in the medium (net flow of particles per unit area in the model) must include a factor for the particle motion due to elasticity.

The form of Maxwell's modified equation for current again demonstrates his field conception and its relationship to the model: total current equals magnetic intensity from rotation minus the electromotive force from elastic distortion. Given that the orientation of the electromotive force is opposite to that of the vortices, the displacement current actually *opens* the closed circuit as required, which again is opposite from the now customary interpretation. Maxwell's form of the expression clearly derives from Model 3. Following along with figure 2.13, if the vortices are conceived as elastic, the total flux density of the particles arises from the rotation of the vortices combined with the displacement effect on the particles from elastic distortion of the vortices. The rotation of the vortices creates translational motion of particles in a conductor in the same direction. The motion of the particles causes elastic distortion of the vortices. The elastic distortion of the vortices, in turn, produces a reactive force on the particles, that is, a restoring force in the opposite direction. Thus, current is represented by the translational motion of the particles minus the effect of the restoring force. The modified equation for current is consistent with T13 and can be coupled with the known equation of continuity for charge to derive an expression linking charge and the electric field, that is, the differential form of the Coulomb law.

Maxwell was now in a position to calculate the velocity of propagation in the model. Because of the additional model constraint:

M6. All displacement is tangential,

he needed to find only the transverse velocity of propagation for the medium. He derived the velocity as equal to the ratio between electrodynamic and electrostatic units, and obtained the value for the constant relating them using the experimental value determined by Weber and Kohlraush. This constant has the dimensions of millimeters per second, a velocity. Maxwell noted that, on converting this number to English units, it is nearly the same value as the velocity of light. What Maxwell said here is significant: "we can scarcely avoid the inference *that light consists in the transverse undulations of the same medium which is the cause of electric and magnetic phenomena*" (ibid., 500, emphasis in the original). That is, the close agreement between the velocities signals more than coincidence. However tempting it was, though, he did "avoid the inference." Note that he was not avoiding the inference that light is an electromagnetic phenomenon here (which clearly he suspected from the outset); he was avoiding an inference about the possible identity of the two media of transmission, the light aether and the electromagnetic aether. Maxwell's reticence reinforces my interpretation: The value of the transverse velocity in the electromagnetic medium was determined *directly and only* from specific suppositions of Model 3, and there were no independent physical grounds on which to assume vortex motion in the light aether. On the then prevailing view, light is a transverse wave in an elastic medium and could not be propagated by the same kind of mechanism as that provided by the model for propagating electromagnetic actions.

Maxwell ended the analysis of Part III by showing how to calculate the electric capacity of a Leyden jar using his analysis of electrostatic force. Part IV applied the whole theory to the rotation of the plane of polarized light by magnetism and showed the direction of rotation to depend on the angular momentum of the molecular vortices, which ties the whole analysis back to the constraints of Part I. With this calculation he established that all the salient constraints were satisfied. Although considerably more work remained to be done in articulating the new representation and finding experimental verification of the propagation of electromagnetic forces, at this point Maxwell had added a new explanatory device to the conceptual and analytical resources of physics—the field representation of forces.

2.3   Discussion: Maxwell's Model-based Reasoning Practices

2.3.1   Maxwell's Modeling versus the Symmetry Argument

Since the Maxwell case is one that has generated significant commentary in the history and philosophy of science, I begin with a brief discussion that situates my analysis with respect to that literature. When I first read through Maxwell's research in electromagnetism in the mid-1970s, I found it surprising how many commentators on this work failed to take seriously what seemed to me to be the generative role of the models developed in the 1861–1862 paper. Maxwell's own comments on "physical analogy" as a method of discovery—in letters, publications, and lectures—were largely dismissed and characterized as at best "merely suggestive" (Heimann 1970), offering "slight" value as heuristic guides (Chalmers 1973, 137),[2] and at worst as dishonest post hoc fabrications (Duhem 1914, 98). In this last case, Duhem claimed that Maxwell had cooked up the physical analogy after the fact and even falsified an equation (see also Duhem 1902), while "the results he obtained were known to him by other means" (1914, 98).

The "known by other means" claim is one that has been made frequently by philosophers. When pressed as to *what* other means, the response is usually that the equations were derived by induction from the experiments, or through consistency arguments pertaining to equations that did not even exist when Maxwell started his research. Certainly experimental results played a key role in Maxwell's analysis, but the process of deriving the equations was not what philosophers usually call "induction." The search for consistency—or the "symmetry account"—explains the derivation of the equations as represented in figure 2.16.

Mark Steiner, in a recent version of the account, states it as "[o]nce the phenomenological laws of Faraday, Coulomb, and Ampere [sic] had been given differential form, Maxwell noted that they contradicted the conservation of electrical charge. . . . Yet, by tinkering with Ampere's [sic] law adding to it the 'displacement current,' Maxwell succeeded in getting the laws actually to imply charge conservation" (Steiner 1989, 458). The "tinkering" is usually interpreted as Maxwell's having noticed that the equation for the magnetic field did not include a contribution from the electric field. This account is often given by physicists as well (see, e.g., Jackson 1962, 177).[3] But what is left out of the symmetry account is the central problem of how Maxwell gave the phenomenological laws differential form in the first place, which leads to a study of his modeling practices and ultimately to a quite different interpretation of the "tinkering" process.

Another common move made by philosophers is to claim that since, in fact, the aether can be eliminated from Maxwell's laws—as it was in Einstein's representation—its role in the development of the theory is

Coulomb Law : $div\,\mathbf{D} = 4\pi\rho$

Ampere Law : $\mathbf{curl\,H} = 4\pi\mathbf{J}$

Faraday Law : $\mathbf{curl\,E} = -\dfrac{\partial\mathbf{B}}{\partial t}$

Absence of free magnetic poles : $div\,\mathbf{B} = 0$

Conservation of charge requires :

Equation of continuity : $div\,\mathbf{J} + \dfrac{\partial\rho}{\partial t} = 0$

Considerations of consistency and symmetry lead to alteration of

Faraday Law : $\mathbf{curl\,E} = -\dfrac{\partial\mathbf{B}}{\partial t} + \dfrac{1}{c^2}\dfrac{\partial\mathbf{E}}{\partial t}$

Figure 2.16
The "symmetry account."

insignificant. This move thus eliminates or reduces the generative role of the models of the aether that Maxwell constructed. Philip Kitcher, for example, claims that the aether was not a "working posit" involved in problem solving, explanation, and prediction, but a "presuppositional posit," which he argues was incorrectly thought to be required to make the claims of the theory true (Kitcher 1993, 174). Since it is not required, it can simply be removed from Maxwell's theory. To the contrary, however, without the working posit of the existence of the aether as a continuum mechanical medium Maxwell could not have derived the equations at all.[4] Eliminating the aether from Maxwell's theory took forty more years of research by several outstanding scientists, most of whom assumed its existence.

I have shown that there are several ways of tracing his reasoning to the models. For example, in the initial analysis of magnetic phenomena, Maxwell focused on a single rotating vortex. But the next phase of the analysis required a medium full of rotating vortices, which produced model constraints leading directly to the introduction of the idle wheel particles with specific characteristics as a way of representing the causal structure of electromagnetic induction. Also, although there are significant sign "errors" in this part of Maxwell's analysis, all but one of these—a minor substitution error—can be seen not to be errors when we view him as reasoning through the constructed models. Additionally, it was only through the models that he came to understand how to represent the energy of the electromagnetic system, which was necessary for rederiving the mathematical representation using generalized dynamics, as he did in the next paper (1864).

In the 1861–1862 paper, Maxwell had said that the causal mechanisms of his models could provide "mechanical explanations" of the phenomena, when understood at a certain level of abstraction. In the *Treatise*, Maxwell said that the problem of "determining the mechanism required to establish a certain species of connexion . . . admits of an infinite number of mechanisms" (1891 470). Although it might have been his original intention to understand the specific mechanisms in the aether that produce electromagnetic forces, the causal mechanisms he was able to construct provide only highly abstract explanations in the form of structural relations; they only specify the *kinds* of mechanical processes that could produce the stresses under examination. They provide no means for picking out which processes actually do produce the stresses. In a later discussion of generalized dynamics, Maxwell likened the situation to that in which the bellringers in the belfry can see only the ropes, not the mechanism that rings the bell (1890b,

783–784). However, the nature of the underlying mechanical forces in the aether remained an open project for Maxwell until his untimely death, and for the physics community for many years thereafter.

We are now in a position to understand the difference between Thomson's and Maxwell's methods of analogy. Thomson's method was to take an existing mathematical representation of a known physical system, such as Fourier's analysis of heat, as an analogical source, construct a mapping of parameters between the source and the target system under investigation, and substitute the parameters for the target system into the source equations, in this case electrostatic parameters. That is, Thomson proceeded directly to the mathematical structures using a formal analogy between the two real-world domains. His is the kind of analogical reasoning process usually discussed in the philosophical and cognitive literatures. What makes Maxwell's 1861–1862 modeling process different is that the analogical sources to be mapped to the domain of electromagnetism were not ready to hand, but had to be constructed. Continuum mechanics did not possess a solved problem with mathematical representations that could be applied directly to the problem. Instead, he constructed a series of models intermediary between the source and target domain, embodying constraints from each domain, and reasoned through these. The derived mathematical expressions capture the structural relations of the models, which represent structural relations common to the target and source domains. Maxwell derived the mathematical structures of the models on the mechanical interpretation, and substituted in the electromagnetic parameters, a move akin to that of Thomson but preceded by a very different reasoning process. For Thomson, the mappings went from a solved problem of one real-world system to another real-world system. Maxwell's mathematical representations were derived from models, for which it does not matter whether the models could exist in their full form as systems in nature; all that matters is that they contain causal structures that are mechanically plausible—feasible mechanisms but not the specific mechanisms giving rise to electromagnetic phenomena.

My interpretation provides a strong case that Maxwell's problem solving was by reasoning through modeling processes that involved constructing several mechanical models taken to represent the causal structure—not the actual causes—of the production and transmission of electric and magnetic forces in a mechanical aether. These models integrate physical and mathematical constraints abstracted from (and held in common with) continuum-mechanical systems, specific machine mechanisms, and electromagnetic systems. The constraints are integrated into a series of *hybrid* models that stand in between the domains. In their mathematical treatment, these common dynamical properties and relationships are separated from the specific systems by means of which they had been made concrete, yielding equations representing both the mechanical and electromagnetic systems.

During the modeling process, Maxwell continually evaluated the models and the inferences he drew from them. The solutions to the subproblems were then integrated into a coherent mathematical representation. As was to be determined only much later, that mathematical representation expresses the dynamical relationships of a *non-Newtonian* dynamical system. That is, the mathematical structure Maxwell derived for electromagnetic phenomena will not map back onto the mechanical source domains used in its creation. This is a highly creative exemplar of model-based reasoning in that a fundamentally new concept was introduced into physics. The modeling process enabled Maxwell to derive the laws of a non-Newtonian system, using Newtonian systems as sources. To explain how will take the rest of this book. As a start, we need to understand an abstractive process I call "abstraction via generic modeling," which I will introduce below with respect to the Maxwell exemplar and discuss more generally in chapter 6.

2.3.2 Abstraction via Generic Modeling

To extend the analysis to Maxwell's subsequent work, the 1864 analysis assumed only that the electromagnetic medium is a generic "connected system," possessing elasticity and thus having energy (see Nersessian 1984). The electromagnetic medium and the light aether are considered the same, and the aether is treated as "a complicated mechanism capable of a vast variety of motion, but at the same time so connected that the motion of one part depends, according to definite relations on the motion of other parts, these motions being communicated by forces arising from the relative displacement of the connected parts, in virtue of their elasticity" (Maxwell 1864, 533). The elasticity of the connected system provides for the time delay in transmission. All that is required is a generic conception of elastic systems as capable of receiving and storing energy. The energy of such a system has two forms: "energy of motion," or kinetic energy, and "energy of tension," or potential energy. Maxwell identified kinetic energy with magnetic polarization and potential energy with electric polarization. Once he had abstracted the appropriate set of general dynamical relations, he could then apply these back to the source domain without the need for any specific model.

The modeling process enabled him to use the powerful representational resources of the mathematics of general dynamics, especially partial differential equations, thereby eliminating the need for an analysis of the actual aether forces underlying electromagnetic phenomena. Briefly (see Buchwald 1985 for a deeper treatment), to describe the motion of a body or systems of bodies in the Newtonian form of mechanics requires calculating the summation of the forces (integration) that each body exerts on the others at each moment. Newton had to invent the mathematical method for doing this kind of analysis, the differential calculus. In the late eighteenth century, Lagrange developed a form of analysis (partial differential equations) that enabled bypassing this infinitesimal summation process and allowed analysis of motion with only finite quantities. One form of his analysis, which became known as potential field analysis, enabled calculation of the forces on a potential system of bodies. For example, one could calculate the force that would arise if one were to put one or more bodies in between an existing two-body system. This is a mathematical result that depends on knowing the potential and kinetic energy (as we now call them) of the system. The potential field does not really exist—the forces arise only if a body were to be placed in between the others. Most importantly, there is no time delay in transmission of the forces. With a time delay, the question of what is going on in the space surrounding bodies and charges must be addressed.

The assumption of this mathematical technique is that the underlying forces in the system are Newtonian action-at-a-distance forces—and indeed it works for mechanical systems: you can rederive Newton's laws in general dynamical form. This method of analysis was a boon to those working on the mechanics of continuous media, such as fluids and elastic substances and things that were thought to be substances such as heat, because to do the analysis the integration way would require summing millions of forces. Instead, one could simply use the macroscopic manifestations to determine the two energy quantities and write the equations of motion for the system. Some of this work was done by analogical mappings, for example, solving the problem for fluids and then mapping directly to heat. Furthermore, continuum mechanics required a representation of directed forces and fields (vectors) that went beyond that needed for gravitational attraction—and Maxwell's analysis of electromagnetism contributed to the development of vector analysis as well. A "curl," for example, is the circulation of forces; a "divergence," the spreading of them.

Maxwell was in the hotbed of this activity in the mid-nineteenth century at Cambridge. But no one had tackled the problem of representing the hypothesized time delay (required for the real field with its own energy and momentum) in transmission of electromagnetic forces. The previous analyses provided only potential field (fictional field) analyses. To solve the representational problem, Maxwell had in essence to determine which macroscopic quantities in the electromagnetic aether (assumed to be a Newtonian mechanical system microscopically) to associate with the two energies, and he did this through the modeling processes I have analyzed. No direct analogies existed, ready to hand to apply. The modeling processes led to a set of partial differential equations for the motion of the system that enabled him to calculate the speed of transmission or the time delay. Once he knew how to represent kinetic and potential energy, he needed only to assume the aether to be a connected system and then rederive the equations of motion using Lagrangian techniques. In the *Treatise* his final derivation was in the new form of vector analysis developed by his colleague William Hamilton. Some of the mathematics needed to represent electromagnetic phenomena existed, and some was codeveloped with the study of electromagnetism. But throughout, Maxwell was assuming these analytical methods were applied to macroscopic phenomena that were created by microscopic Newtonian forces.

Throughout his reasoning processes, Maxwell abstracted from the specific mechanism represented in the model to the mathematical form of that *kind* of mechanism, in other words, of the generic dynamical structure. This move is at the heart of the disagreement between Maxwell and Thomson, who never did accept Maxwell's mathematical representation because it does not derive from a real-world solution. Maxwell's own position was that his field equations were not any worse off than Newton's law of gravitation, since that, too, had been formulated without any knowledge of the specific underlying causal mechanisms. In Maxwell's time, generalized dynamics and Newtonian mechanics were thought to be coextensive. What we know today that Maxwell did not is that many different kinds of dynamical systems can be formulated in the mathematics of generalized dynamics, including relativity and quantum mechanics. Electrodynamical systems are not the same kind of dynamical system as Newtonian systems. What he abstracted through the generic modeling process is a representation of the general dynamical properties and relationships for electromagnetism. The abstract laws, when applied to electromagnetism, yield the laws of a dynamical system that is nonmechanical—that is, laws that do not map back onto the mechanical domains used in their construction. Maxwell's equations yield fundamentally new kinds of models.

Failing to follow the well-known dictum of Einstein,[5] many have dismissed Maxwell's deeds in the philosophical, historical, and science literature as noted above; for in dismissing the 1861–1862 modeling practices, we are left with no evidence in Maxwell's papers, drafts, and correspondence as to what "other means" he might have employed. By examining his "deeds," however, we find there is a remarkable harmony between word and deed in Maxwell's work. As with Einstein and Newton, Maxwell is one scientist from whom we can learn a great deal about the nature of scientific practices by heeding both his words and his deeds. I have argued that Maxwell constructed the mathematical representation for the electromagnetic field concept through an incremental modeling process that involved creating and reasoning by means of a series of interrelated models so as to satisfy empirical, theoretical, and mathematical constraints. In concluding the chapter, I turn to consider the model-based reasoning somewhat divorced from the content to find clues as to what makes it productive in conceptual innovation. The next section also serves to summarize the Maxwell exemplar for those who have opted to skip most of the details.

2.3.3 Model-based Reasoning in Conceptual Innovation

The three models Maxwell created are interpretations of the target phenomena constructed to satisfy constraints drawn from the target domain of electricity and magnetism, the source domains of continuum mechanics and machine mechanics, and from the constructed models themselves. These hybrid models stand in between the target and source domain and provide contexts in which to reason and draw inferences that include mathematical equations and physical hypotheses. Each model iteration was reasonable and contextually well motivated. Each model led to insights into and elaboration of the constraints of the target domain, to a mathematical representation of some of the target phenomena, and to further problems whose representational solutions were provided by the affordances of the model itself. The end result provided a radical reconceptualization of the domain of electromagnetism.

In the course of his analysis Maxwell discussed the nature of the properties and relations in the models he constructed, drew schematic representations of features of the models, expressed imagined simulations, and provided instructions for how others could visualize and imagine animating the visual representations in their own reasoning. Although he did not state directly that he, himself, was visualizing or simulating motion of the medium and mechanisms in his own thought, it is hard to "avoid the inference" that he would have been. Clearly his own accounts of physical analogy and various forms of mathematical representation in this paper and in numerous other settings lead the interpretation in that direction. Maxwell's writings are peppered with talk of "mental operations" in physical and mathematical reasoning. One particularly nice expression of his reflections appears in an article in the journal *Nature* about the new mathematical formalism, Hamilton's method of quaternions, that Maxwell used in the *Treatise*: "It does not . . . encourage the hope that mathematicians may give their minds a holiday, by transferring all their work to their pens. It calls upon us at every step to form a mental image of the geometrical features represented by the symbols so that in studying geometry in this way, we have our minds engaged with geometrical ideas, and are not permitted to fancy ourselves geometers when we are only arithmeticians" (Maxwell 1873, 137). My contention is that the evidence weighs in favor of Maxwell's mind being "engaged with the geometrical ideas" while making inferences from the models.

On my interpretation, the general categories of reasoning in Maxwell's modeling processes include (not ordered): abstractive, simulative, adaptive, and evaluative. Figure 2.17 provides a schematic representation of his reasoning processes that serves to highlight the interactions among the target domain, source domains, and the constructed models.

Abstractive reasoning includes limiting case extrapolation, idealization, generalization, and what I call "abstraction via generic modeling," which will be discussed below. Simulative reasoning comprises making inferences through manipulating a model by animation, such as imagining the consequences of the motion of vortices on the idle wheels and vice versa. Conceiving of the vortices side by side in motion in Model 1 (see figure 2.10) led Maxwell to recognize that friction between adjacent vortices would stop their motion. His inference pertaining to a general notion of friction led him to adapt the model by introducing the idle wheel particles. The adaptations he made were in response to both problems with the models and his altered understanding of the target problems (represented in figure 2.17 by target[+] and target[++]) derived from them. The latter includes making inferences to new constraints provided by the earlier model(s), as when he inferred what would happen to the vortices when the idle wheel particles are in motion in Model 2 or undergo a slight translational motion in place in Model 3. His evaluation of the models generally proceeded from considerations of whether selected features of the models were of the *same kind* with respect to salient dimensions of the target phenomena, such as with respect to the structure of causal relations between electricity and magnetism in Model 2. These evaluations led to adaptations, as in the

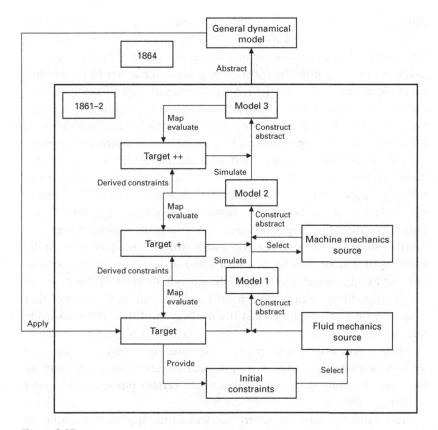

Figure 2.17
Maxwell's modeling process.

above instance where Maxwell recognized that Model 1 is not of the same kind as an electrodynamic system because the model could not sustain motion given the friction between vortices. His evaluative considerations included goodness of fit to the constraints, empirical implications, mathematical implications, and explanatory power. In constructing the models Maxwell used domain knowledge, knowledge of abstract principles, and knowledge of how to make appropriate abstractions. This knowledge was represented in various informational formats, including verbal, mathematical, and visual.

A key feature of the models is that for one to reason with them as representing the electromagnetic phenomena, they must be construed as lacking specificity with respect to the mechanisms creating the stresses in the medium. The source domains served the function of providing constraints and generative principles for building the models, which in turn are the objects of reasoning. The models provide specific mechanisms, but these need to be understood at a sufficient level of abstraction so as to enable recognizing how the constraints apply and transfer to the electromagnetic domain. That is, the models are specific but in the reasoning context they are taken to represent generic processes. Consider, for example, the analysis of electromagnetic induction on Model 2. In reasoning with this model, one is to understand that the causal relational structure between the vortices and the idle wheel particles is maintained but not the specific causal mechanism of vortices and particles. Indeed, the specific mechanism is highly implausible as a fluid dynamical system in nature. The specific mechanism need not be realistic, however, since what it represents is a causal structure, not a specific cause. In solving the various representational problems, Maxwell treated the causal structure as separated from the specific physical systems by means of which it had been made concrete. The vortex–idle wheel mechanism should not be seen as the cause of electromagnetic induction. It represents only the causal structure of that unspecified underlying process in the medium, and the inferences made refer to that structure. Any mechanism that could represent the causal structure would suffice. The specific mechanism is treated generically, in the way a spring or a pendulum could be treated generically as representing the class of simple harmonic oscillators for certain purposes and under certain conditions.

The relation between the generic model and the specific representation used is similar to that between type and instance. Generality in representation is achieved by the reasoner interpreting the components of the representation as referring to object, property, relation, or behavior types rather than instances of these. Representing generic mechanisms by concrete processes gave Maxwell an embodied object to reason about, but the reasoning context demanded that specific physical hypotheses belonging to the source domains not be imported to the analysis of the target problem. Consider the instance of introducing the idle wheels. As we saw, Model 2 is a hybrid constructed from two source domains: fluid dynamics and machine mechanics. To recognize the potential mechanism and to combine salient entities and processes from two disparate domains requires that these be considered at a sufficient level of generality.

Similar abstractive reasoning enabled Maxwell to identify the energy components of an electromagnetic system and, in the 1864 analysis, move directly to a general dynamical formulation without the specifics of the 1861–1862 models. Figure 2.18 illustrates my interpretation of Maxwell's reasoning.

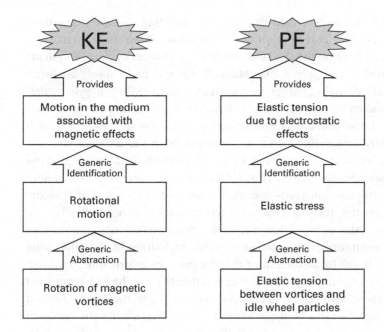

Figure 2.18
Identifying energy components via generic modeling.

In the 1864 analysis Maxwell treated the aether as a generic elastic medium whose constraints could be satisfied by many specific mechanical instantiations. Elastic systems can receive and store energy in two forms, kinetic energy (motion) and potential energy (tension). Schematically, for Models 1 through 3, kinetic energy is associated with the rotation of vortices, which can be abstracted to a generic notion of "rotational motion," which then in the general dynamical analysis is identified with the motion in the medium associated with magnetic effects. On Model 3, potential energy is associated with elastic tension between the vortices and the idle wheel particles, which can be abstracted to a generic notion of "elastic stress," which in the general dynamical analysis is identified with elastic tension due to electrostatic effects. Interestingly, and adding plausibility to my interpretation, vestiges of the earlier specific mechanical model can be shown to have remained in his 1864 thinking; this created a problem with the current and charge equations, which would take us too far afield to discuss here (see Nersessian 2001, 2002c).

On my interpretation of Maxwell's reasoning, we have a plausible answer to the puzzle of creativity in conceptual change posed earlier. In this case the puzzle is: If Maxwell really did derive the mathematical representation of the electromagnetic field through the modeling processes described, how is it possible that by making analogies from Newtonian mechanical domains he constructed the laws of a non-Newtonian dynamical system? The answer lies in seeing that Maxwell did not make direct analogies between the domains. Rather, he constructed intermediary, hybrid models that embodied constraints from both Newtonian sources and the electro- magnetic target domain. Abstractive processes, especially generic model- ing, enabled integrating selective constraints from the different domains because they were considered at a level of generality that eliminated the domain-specific differences. Thus a fundamentally new kind of represen- tational structure emerged—one that abstracted the notion of "mecha- nism" from the analysis, creating a representation of a nonmechanical, dynamical system. The mathematical representation derived in this manner provides no information about the specific realization of the underlying system. Maxwell himself assumed that the underlying structure comprised mechanical interactions in the aether and that the laws he had formulated acted as constraints on any acceptable mechanism. In this he saw himself as following the same strategy Newton had in formulating the universal law of gravitation: "investigat[ing] the forces with which bodies act on each other in the first place, before attempting to explain *how* that force is transmitted" (Maxwell 1890b, emphasis in the original). And, indeed, we could construct a similar story for how Newton used model-based rea- soning and abstraction via generic modeling in his derivation of this law. As we know, the history of attempts to specify the "how" in both the Newtonian and Maxwellian cases led to further major conceptual changes in physics.

My interpretation of Maxwell as reasoning through model construction, manipulation, and adaptation assumes certain cognitive capacities for car- rying out such reasoning, namely, simulative, analogical, and imagistic modes of thinking. I will turn to a discussion of the cognitive basis of model-based reasoning after first developing a parallel exemplar of such practices in a case of solving a more mundane problem as exhibited in a protocol study.

3 Model-based Reasoning Practices: Protocol Study Exemplar

The whole of science is nothing more than a refinement of everyday thinking. It is for this reason that the critical thinking of a physicist cannot possibly be restricted to the examination of concepts of his own specific field. He cannot proceed without considering critically a much more difficult problem, the problem of analyzing the nature of everyday thinking.
—Albert Einstein, *Physics and Reality*

This chapter presents a case of creative (P-creative) model-based reasoning in an instance of conceptual innovation and change for an individual. At the beginning of the protocol session, S2's concept of spring did not include the central notion that the stretch of a spring takes place through a twisting force, namely, torsion. Although S2's conceptual innovation is modest, his model-based reasoning practices that led to it provide an instance of highly creative problem solving that exhibits many of the features of the Maxwell case. Since the subject matter is less complex and the reasoning requires less knowledge to follow, it can substitute as an exemplar for those who find the Maxwell case tough going. Additionally, it serves as support for the continuum hypothesis of cognitive-historical analysis. Juxtaposing the two cases serves to exhibit the commonalities between innovative scientific reasoning and creative reasoning in more ordinary problem solving.

The protocol study is both richer and more impoverished than the Maxwell case. It is richer in detail in that we can assume that the steps along the way are recorded and follow in the actual order of the reasoning. S2 sketches his models and gestures their simulations. Given that the subject attempts to report all thinking, there are frequent references to visualizations and simulative imaginings that we can only infer in the Maxwell case. The protocol is impoverished compared with the Maxwell case in the artificial nature of the problem situation. We do, however, have some information about S2's background that helps one understand the origin of the analogical source domains he used in this context. Finally, S2 is not an expert in the domain of springs—or in physics. Recall, however, that Maxwell, too, though an expert mathematical physicist, was something of a novice in electricity and magnetism when he began working on the problem of constructing a unified mathematical representation. He used his expertise in continuum mechanics in solving the problem. Similarly, S2 used his expertise in topology in solving the problem. They each drew from source domains in which they had deep knowledge and had done significant prior problem solving using the practices they had acquired from their respective communities.

3.1 Protocol Records and Analysis

For those unfamiliar with protocol experiments, it will be useful to highlight, briefly, some features of the records used in protocol analysis in comparison with historical records. In a think-aloud protocol experiment, participants are provided with a problem to solve and are asked to verbalize—and possibly to sketch—their thoughts as they occur, while they are video- or audiotaped. Both historical data and protocol data can provide primary data for hypotheses about the nature of cognitive processes in problem solving (see also Klahr and Simon 1999; Feist and Gorman 1998). Potential differences and similarities in the two kinds of data cluster around the following issues: (1) when and how the data are recorded, (2) the granularity of the data, (3) the problem situation in which the data are produced, and (4) the nature of the practices in which the data are produced and recorded.

On the customary interpretation (Ericsson and Simon 1984), a think-aloud problem-solving protocol is taken to provide "a direct trace" (220) of the concurrent thinking. The presumption is that the protocol provides direct evidence of the information heeded, the structure of the problem solving (or sequence of steps), and the strategies employed. It has been shown in several experiments that verbalization, per se, affects at most the speed of the problem-solving process (ibid., 63–106). Verbalization is held not to interfere with the nature of the ongoing reasoning if carried out in the prescribed manner. This assumes that the problem solver does not try to explain his or her reasoning, but rather reports what he or she is attending to, remembering, and so forth. Although producing a concurrent narrative might involve some modality change, such as conveying an image in words, it does not require additional intellectual work such as constructing an argument to persuade someone else or an explanation to help someone else understand. Since the record is concurrent for protocol data, the claim that the problem solution was "by some other means" would be more difficult to make. The problem-solving protocols are designed to make reasoning public.

With historical records it is unknown exactly how close to the thinking they were recorded. Laboratory notebooks and diaries are likely candidates for records close to the original thinking (Gooding 1990; Tweney 1985, 1989; Holmes 1981, 1985), correspondence varies in proximity, and publications are likely to be the farthest removed. Notebook and diary entries made closer to the thinking are more likely to recall the information heeded and the sequence, or temporal order, of thinking, as has been demonstrated with studies on retrospective verbalization (Ericsson and Simon 1984 148–159). However, as all historians know, every piece of recorded data needs to be treated as a reconstruction by its author. Thus, as noted in chapter 2, analysis of a historical problem-solving episode requires making a case on the basis of convergent evidence from a number and variety of sources.

The objective of a think-aloud protocol is to record as a fine-grained thought-by-thought record of the concurrent thinking as the subject is capable of expressing. Although cognitive scientists sometimes seem to treat protocols as akin to volt-meter registrations, it would be mistaken to think of the protocol record as complete registrations of cognitive processes. For one thing, people are not perfectly aware of what they are thinking, and there are clearly limits on what can be heeded at any one time, both of which can cause gaps in a sequence or seemingly unmotivated changes in direction. Thus protocols are claimed to provide only *a subset* of the problem-solving processes (Ericsson and Simon 1984, 109–167). With historical records, "fine-grained" is most applicable to notebooks and diaries, and the granularity depends largely on the individual. These kinds of records range from highly detailed accounts in which the scientist has attempted to record concurrent thinking processes to less detailed notes meant to capture processes having occurred in close proximity to scanty records that are only cryptic reminders to the researcher.

With respect to the extent of the record, in a think-aloud protocol, an actual problem solution is either obtained or not in a session lasting not more than a couple of hours. In historical cases, where there is a problem solution, it often emerged over days, months, or even years, providing an extensive record comprising many kinds of documents—of successes and failures—that can assist the cognitive-historical researcher. In both instances interpolation and interpretation are required. In the case of protocols, these are made on the basis of the researcher's preexisting models of cognitive processes and of what knowledge the researcher expects the subject to possess. Typically there is only scant information about the background and knowledge of the participant. In the historical cases, there are usually significantly more data to draw upon for interpolating, and there are far greater resources for determining the intellectual, social, and cultural contexts of the problem solving.

Finally, for data to be meaningful, they need to be understood within the context of the assumptions employed in the practices that inform their production and collection. There is an extensive and well-known philosophical literature in the twentieth century (starting with Hanson 1958, Feyerabend 1962, Kuhn 1962) that has argued convincingly that observation always takes place within the context of some theoretical assumptions, whether tacit or explicit. All data are collected and selected in accordance with background presuppositions (Shapere 1982). I have noted above some of the assumptions made in the practices of protocol experiments and of historical interpretation. All data are produced within social and cultural contexts, which requires heeding, for instance, the conventions of a practice such as writing. A published paper participates in a set of community practices and is intended to advance understanding within that community. Since it is derivative from a set of practices, it also provides insight into how understanding is achieved in that community. In the case of protocol reports, the experimental situation itself sets up a social practice in which the subject and the experimenter participate. One explicit convention of this practice is for the subject to report in a way consistent with the instructions—not to explain or justify, but simply to express thoughts as they occur. Protocol records can be transcribed so as to focus just on the words, but visual records created or gestures used can be part of the analysis. An implicit convention is for the subject to convey what he is thinking in a way that he thinks the experimenter will find meaningful. So, for example, there are bound to be differences in the language used to report a thought if a subject is a physicist and knows he is talking to another physicist or to a nonscientist.

The protocol analyzed in this exemplar derives from an audiotape, which has been transcribed in 22 pages, and a videotape. I have used the method of "verbal analysis" (Chi 1997) in coding and analyzing it. This method is more flexible and better suited to my purposes than formal "protocol analysis" (Ericsson and Simon 1984), which assumes that the aim is to build a production-system type computational model.

Chi (1997) describes eight steps in coding verbal data:

1. reducing or sampling the protocols.
2. segmenting the reduced or sampled protocols.
3. developing a coding scheme or formalism.
4. operationalizing evidence in the coded protocols to provide a mapping to the code/formalism.
5. depicting the mapped formalism.
6. seeking patterns in the mapped formalism.
7. interpreting the pattern(s).
8. repeating the process, possibly coding at a different grain size (optional).

There is no need to reduce or sample the S2 protocol since the entire reasoning process is to be analyzed. The segmentation is according to reasoning chains related to each of the four models the subject created. Since the Maxwell modeling process had been analyzed in terms of the constraints that needed to be satisfied in model construction, evaluation, and modification, and in terms of his use of analogies, visualizations, and abstractive processes, my coding focused on these in the S2 protocol.[1]

3.2   Exemplar 2: S2 and the Concept of Spring

This second case study derives from a think-aloud problem-solving protocol experiment designed by John Clement (1989).[2] The problem posed is as follows:

A weight is hung from a spring. The original spring is replaced with a spring: made of the same kind of wire; with the same number of coils; but with coils that are twice as wide in diameter. Will the spring stretch from its natural length more, less, or the same amount under the same weight? (Assume the mass of the spring is negligible compared to the mass of the weight.) Why do you think so? (Clement 1989, 342)

It is possible to arrive at the correct answer to the first question of whether the second spring will stretch more without being able to give a correct answer to the question of why, as did some of the problem solvers. The subjects were faculty and advanced graduate students in scientific or technical fields, including physics, mathematics, and computer science. Only those in physics might be considered to have expertise with springs, but all had facility with advanced methods of problem solving in scientific or technical fields. In all there were eleven protocols, most of which exhibited forms of model-based reasoning. Among them, however, the "S2" case

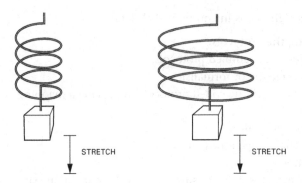

Figure 3.1
Clement's figures accompanying the text of the problem.

is unique in that, as Clement noted, it led to "the invention of a new model of hidden mechanisms in the spring that [the subject] had not observed" (Clement 1989, 378). At the beginning of the problem-solving session, S2's concept of spring did not contain the notion of torsion, and he understood the stretch of a spring as due to bending and flexibility in the wire of the spring. At the end of the session he had come to understand that the stretch of a spring involves a force, torsion, which maintains the uniform stretch of the spring through twisting rather than bending. That is, in the process of finding a satisfactory explanation, S2 had to construct a novel representation for himself of how a spring works. Of the subjects in the protocol study, S2 was the only case of a (P-creative) conceptual innovation during the reasoning process. The other (three) subjects who solved the problem correctly and who included a correct explanation already had the notion of torsion or twist as part of their representation.

Clement's initial (1989) analysis of the protocol focused on a process he calls modeling via bridging analogies; his later analyses have looked at the role of visualization and simulative gesturing (Clement 1994, 2003). He characterized the process of bridging analogies as that in which intermediate analogies are produced by the problem solver between a target and a "farther" analogy. He describes S2 as producing a series of progressively more adequate models "via a successive refinement process of hypothesis generation, evaluation, and modification or rejection" (1989, 358). My analysis of the protocol concurs with his account as a general characterization, but specifies in detail how the "hypothesis generation" takes place through various abstractive processes and simulation, evaluation, and adaptation of models constructed to satisfy target, source, and model constraints. The protocol was captured on audio- and videotape. Since I have only had access to the transcriptions and drawings, when I discuss visualization and simulation in the modeling I am relying on Clement's (2003, 2005) accounts of S2's gestures during the process and his answers to my queries about specific sections of the videotape as I was writing this chapter.

3.3 S2's Problem Situation

As in the Maxwell exemplar, S2's problem solving is embedded in a community of background knowledge, including analytical practices and conceptual resources. Unlike that case, it is not possible to construct a detailed account of these factors for S2 from existing records, in part because of human subject research regulations, and in part because protocol experiments do not usually collect such data. According to Clement, S2 has a Ph.D. in a technical field, had taken some physics courses, and had passed comprehensive examinations in mathematics in the area of topology, though he is not a mathematician. As we will see, it turned out that his expertise in topology proved to be significant to the way he solved the problem. Another dissimilarity between this exemplar and the Maxwell one is that S2 did not pose his problem or inherit it from his intellectual community; rather it is an arbitrary problem posed to him in an artificial context. Clearly, however, S2 found the problem intellectually challenging and became determined to figure out what he felt he did not understand about the stretch of a spring. He even rejected Clement's offers to end the session before he had an explanation since it went on for quite a long time. I take his behavior as indicating that it transformed into a problem *for him*—one that he needed to solve—not just one given to him. The problem-solving episode also was embedded in a set of practices around collecting think-aloud protocols, which include instructions to speak thoughts aloud as they occur and not to analyze these or offer retrospective explanations. Finally, S2 likely knew that Clement is trained in physics and is a researcher in cognitive science and physics education. Although we cannot say decidedly, this knowledge might have formed an important part of the problem situation in that such knowledge could have framed how S2 reported his thoughts, for example, his choice of language.

3.4 S2's Modeling Processes

3.4.1 Model 1: Flexible Rod

The given initial target problem constraints stated explicitly include:

T1. The wire is of the same kind.

T2. The number of coils is constant.

T3. The coil width varies.

T4. The mass of the spring is negligible.

T5. The added weight is constant.

An implicit constraint, given the dynamical situation of the problem, is:

T6. The wire is flexible.

S2 quickly produced a flexible rod as an initial analogical model. After expressing some concern that he "might have real problems conceptualizing it," he stated that "it occurs to me that a spring is nothing but a rod wound up" (005).[3] Although he did not say directly how he arrived at the rod model, I take this and other statements as evidence that he mentally simulated fully extending the spring, which produces a straight wire.[4] On my interpretation, then, Model 1 is derived from a simulation of S2's representation of the target object.

S2 was now in a position to use what we might call "the domain of rods or rodlike objects" as an analogical source domain from which to make inferences about how the behaviors of a rod might compare with those of a spring. He immediately recognized that something is wrong with the proposal, because a spring and a rod do not stretch the same way. We can see that the rod model satisfies constraints T1 through T6 by mapping the increase in coil width to increase in rod length. However, in the dynamic case the rod "would—droop like that and its slope steadily increase as you—went away from the point of attachment, whereas in a spring the slope of the spiral is constant" (005). Clement (2003, 2) notes that as S2 was describing the droop, he traced the downward curve in the air.

This intuition quite plausibly derived from a mental simulation, either partially assisted by or exhibited to the interviewer through his tracing, in the air, of a rod as it bends (see again figure 3.2). From the simulation one can infer that the slope of the rod is greater at positions closer to the weight. At first S2 was not sure that this intuition was correct, and spent several minutes trying to convince himself of it. He expressed that he was going to "try to visualize it or imagine what would happen" and concluded that the answer to the problem is that the spring with wider coils would stretch more. He commented on this imaginative experience as "not really a visualization, it's a kind of kinesthetic sense that somehow a bigger spring is looser." The "kinesthetic sense" led to the correct conclusion that the wider spring would stretch farther, but S2 did not have an explanation for

Original Model

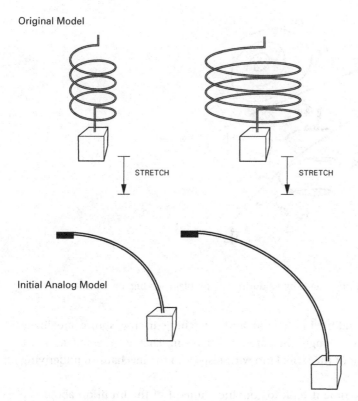

Initial Analog Model

Figure 3.2
My drawing of the spring-to-rod transformation.

why this would be so. At this point he formulated *his* own problem, the one that would guide the rest of the protocol and keep him working until he had reached a satisfactory answer, even when told by the interviewer that he could stop before that point:

Why does a spring stretch?—Why does it stretch?—Does it stretch because a spring bends? Why does a spring stretch at all—come to think of it, what does a spring do? (007)

It is evident, here, that S2's initial concept of spring did not include a representation of the mechanism of stretch, even though his intuitions about springs had led him to the correct answer. We, of course, do not know exactly what his experiences with springs might have been, but his strong kinesthetic intuitions indicate that he had some (perhaps with the ubiquitous "slinky"?). We can, however, infer that S2 realized

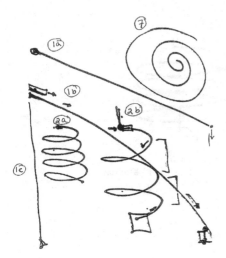

Figure 3.3
Sheet 1 of drawings made by S2 during the problem solving, in context.

here that bending in the rod and stretching in the spring are likely not to occur through the same mechanism. That is, the rod and the spring are not of the same kind with respect to the mechanism underlying their dynamics.

During the time it took to convince himself of the intuition about the constant slope of the stretching spring, he drew pictures of rods and springs "to help fix [them] visually" (007) (figure 3.3).

It is important for later in my analysis to note here that that his drawing of the rod (figure 3.3, 1a) has it rotated at approximately forty-five degrees in the vertical plane. I have separated out these figures to make their features easier to see (figure 3.4).

From the perspective of figure 3.4A, a rod fixed at the top would clearly bend with increasing slope ("droop" as in figure 3.4B) under a constant weight, and, as he noted after drawing the springs on the sheet (see figure 3.3, 2a, 2b), it would "just plain flop" (figure 3.4C) if it were not fixed at the top.

As he drew the spring (figure 3.5A) he noted that it, on the other hand, would be free to "pivot" (adding the indication of the pivot to figure 3.5B) and "something about that sustains the angle—of the coil" (021).

As he talked he drew arrows, annotating the original figures to indicate motion, and, for the spring, he drew bars indicating that the slope is the

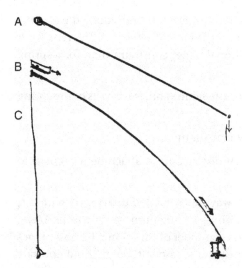

Figure 3.4
S2's rod model drawings 1(a)–1(c).

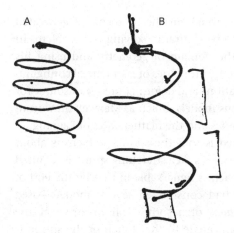

Figure 3.5
S2's spring model drawings 2(a)–2(b).

same for different parts of the spring as it stretches. At various points he expressed that he was imagining and using his "physical intuition" (009) as the basis for his account of the motion, and he made gestures accompanying his descriptions of the motion.

At the end of this segment of reasoning with and about the flexible rod model, S2 had the understanding that springiness is different from bendability and inferred the additional target constraint that, for a spring with wire of negligible weight:

T7. The slope of the spring remains the same at different parts of the spring during stretching under the weight

which does not match the model constraint:

M1. The rod's slope increases with distance from attachment point as it bends under the weight.

This difference is indicated in the way he annotated drawings (figure 3.3, 1b, 2b) with arrows and brackets. Thus, for the purposes of this problem, the rod cannot be considered a *generic* model of the spring, because it violates the derived constraint for the dynamic case. Although S2 did not state this explicitly, I infer that he understood that if two objects are of the same kind regarding a mechanism of distortion, they should be alike in whether the distortion is or is not uniform throughout the extent of the object.

3.4.1.1 Geometrical Insights I Throughout the protocol, S2 generated geometrical insights that proved to be central in solving the problem. In so doing, he was drawing from the domain of geometry and using his expertise in topology—the study of the properties of geometrical configurations under continuous transformations and deformations—as a source for constructing spontaneous analogous models, much as Maxwell drew from his expertise in continuum mechanics and the mathematics of Lagrangian dynamics. What needs to be noted is that the spring problem is about *dynamics*, that is, an analysis of the forces on a stretching spring is required to answer the problem. S2's approach is remarkable in that by the end of the problem-solving episode, he had constructed several models based on various *topological transformations* of a spring coil to arrive at the dynamical insight that the constant angle in the stretch of the spring is due to torsion or a twisting force, rather than bending.[5] Since he used geometry as a source domain for generating constraints in model construction, I will discuss the significant geometrical insights that arose from each model.

Before constructing Model 2, S2 generated two insights that would later be revisited in finding the satisfactory model (023). First, after stating that he was "visualizing a single coil of a spring," he inferred that "a single coil wrapped around is the same as a whole spring," which led him to hypothesize that it might be possible to reason just about a single coil as a limiting case of a spring. He did not pursue this possibility here, however, because in this problem context the hypothesis led him directly back to the "straightened spring [rod] model." That is, a single coil will also unwind into a rod. Second, he speculated that "the coil is an accidental feature" which led to the inference "surely you could coil a spring in squares, let's say, and it wouldn't—it would behave more or less the same" (023). That is, the actual shape of the spring coils should not cause a significant difference in the stretching behavior. Later, and in a different context, these intuitions would play a role in his inference that torsion is what keeps the spring slope constant. In the present context, however, the second insight led to two unsatisfactory models that are imaginary hybrid constructions of the spring and the rod. These hybrids derive from his attempt to integrate the slope constraint T7 with the fact that a spring has repeating coils. In each case the model is composed of repeating flexible rods. So, it appears that in entertaining the single coil, S2 realized that Model 1 will result from either a single coil spring or a repeating coil spring, and now he wondered if the fact that a spring has several repeating segments was salient after all. In constructing the next two models he, thus, entertained as possibly relevant the constraint

T8. A spring consists of repeating segments.

The next two models he constructed were imaginary explorations of ways to modify the initial model in attempting to satisfy this constraint (sheet 2 drawings 3 and 4, shown in figure 3.6).

3.4.2 Model 2: Zigzag Wire
At the start of this reasoning segment, S2 stated: "Ah! From squares, visually I suddenly get a kind of zigzag spring rather than a coiled spring" (023) and drew a picture of the zigzag model (shown in figure 3.7).

He then stressed that the drawing was to be viewed as a "2-dimensional spring," not as a "profile of a 3-dimensional spring" (023). What he claimed to have visualized is a hybrid model—one constructed with features of both springs and rods. It is not clear why he limited the view to two dimensions, but this restricted significantly the inferences made from it. He endowed this hybrid rod–spring model with new constraints:

M2. The rods are rigid.
M3. All bending is at the joints.

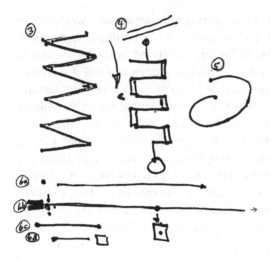

Figure 3.6
Sheet 2 of drawings made by S2 during the problem solving, in context.

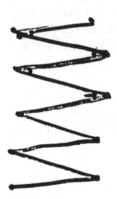

Figure 3.7
S2's zigzag model drawing.

He quickly saw, however, that in the dynamic case the zigzag fails to satisfy an implicit target constraint that this model had allowed him to recognize: "the springiness of a spring—the real spring—is a distributed springiness" (023), or:

T9. The distribution of stretch is uniform.

This constraint is actually just a reformulation of the earlier slope constraint T7. Here, however, S2 appears to be trying to draw on knowledge

of physics in making the inference that bending at the joints is incompatible with the uniform distribution of stretch in the target case, as is indicated by his searching for the correct terminology: "I, er, forgot the word
for that—tensile strength?" (023).

S2, thus, rejected Model 2 because for the zigzag, all the "springiness" is
at the joints whereas for the spring, it is distributed along it. This violation
of type is another version of that used to reject Model 1, that is, distortion
of stretching is uniform throughout the spring, but is not uniform in the
zigzag model.

3.4.3   Model 3: Rigid Connector Wire

S2 constructed Model 3 in an attempt to integrate the target constraint of
"distributed springiness" T9 into Model 2. S2 claimed to first visualize
before drawing what he considered a potentially satisfactory mechanism:
inserting connecting segments of rigid vertical rods between the angles of
the two-dimensional zigzags (figure 3.8).

In this model the horizontal rods are flexible, as is consistent with
the rod in Model 1. S2 assured himself that the rigid connector model
has "springiness" by imagining "kinesthetically" (025) pulling it, noting—
and annotating the drawing with an arrow—that as one imagines stretching it and letting go, "it bounces up and down," as does a spring. However,
if the spring and the Model 3 are to be of the same kind, the stretch needs
to be uniformly distributed. S2 then came back to the thought that perhaps
repeating does not matter and that it should be possible to consider just

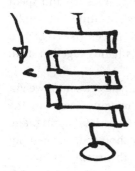

Figure 3.8
S2's rigid connector wire drawing.

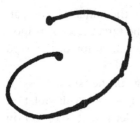

Figure 3.9
S2's first single coil drawing.

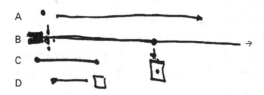

Figure 3.10
S2's drawings of a series of rods.

one segment, just as one can consider a single segment of the spring. During these considerations he drew a single spring coil (figure 3.9).

He did not state directly here that a single segment would unwind into a rod, but he began a line of reasoning that recognizes this implicitly since it led him back to thinking again about why Model 1 would not work.

During this process he drew a series of rods (see figure 3.10) and spent considerable time considering his "physical imagistic intuition" (025) about the slope of the bending rod, imagining what it feels like to bend a rod. (Clement [2005, 3] observes that S2 placed his hands together as in gripping a rod and then moved them slightly.)

He then considered what would happen by varying placement of weight along the rod and then (after taking a phone call) "imagined" moving the weight along both a rod of various lengths and a "massless" spring, and "taking it to the limiting case" (027) of an extremely short rod. Throughout this reasoning process he continued to refer to the spring stretch as "bending." This was followed by a period of reflecting on whether a spring with wider coils is the same as a longer spring, that is, one with more coils but the same length of wire. Here he expressed the concern that the fact that a spring consists of coils "just seems geometrically irrelevant" (041), but did not elaborate on what he meant. However, it does provide a clue that at this point he began to draw explicitly again from the source domain of geometry. At the end of this reasoning segment he expressed more confidence in his answer that the spring with wider coils would stretch more, but he was still bothered by the "anomaly" (045) that the constant slope constraint of the spring is violated by straightening it into a rod.

3.4.3.1 Geometrical Insights II S2 next claimed to have a visual image that he described as "expresses what I am thinking" (049). This was followed by the thought that with the rod one "is always measuring in the vertical—maybe somehow the way the—the coiled spring unwinds, makes for a different frame of reference" (049). This is a highly significant geometrical insight because it appears to have started him thinking and visualizing three-dimensionally. Recall that earlier he qualified his representations of the spring-as-rod models as being two-dimensional. This shift in perspective would lead, though not immediately, to Model 4, an open, three-dimensional single coil oriented in the horizontal plane, which affords a different kind of simulation of stretching. In the current context, however, he first spent some time again reassuring himself that the spring has constant slope, explicitly calling on mathematical knowledge of differentials. This reasoning segment began with S2 trying to imagine the inverse action of winding up the rod into a spring while maintaining the changing slope of the rod. But he recognized this would not be possible if the wound-up rod were truly coiled like a spring. He then noted that straightening the spring, as in the rod model, of course removes the curvature, and observed that for the spring "all its curvature is sort of horizontal—or near horizontal as the coils curl around" (055). Again, this indicates a shift in his attention to the horizontal plane in which a three-dimensional spring stretches.

He then spent some time thinking about the geometry of unwinding the coil and the differences between spirals and helices, drawing a picture of a flat spiral (figure 3.11) and comparing it with his earlier drawing on that sheet of an unwinding spring (see figure 3.5B).

The differences between how S2 was conceiving of a spiral and a helix are not explained, but in the context, the fact that a helix is a three-dimensional geometrical figure seems significant. Again recall that the rod models were two-dimensional figures and their bend or stretch is in the vertical plane. The contrast he appears to be making is that between a two-dimensional figure, such as the flat spiral he drew, and a three-dimensional figure that would have a horizontal component to the stretch. The geometrical insight segment generated a target constraint that was central in constructing Model 4:

T10. The coiling of a spring is in the horizontal plane.

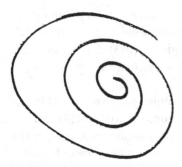

Figure 3.11
S2's drawing of a spiral.

Once he had achieved this perspective, S2 noted that what he meant by
"spiral" earlier actually should be "helix."

3.4.4   Model 4: Horizontal Coil

These geometrical considerations were followed by an extended segment
in which S2 expressed greater confidence in his answer that the wider
spring would stretch more, but even greater frustration that he could not
explain why. However, he rejected the interviewer's offer to end the protocol session, saying "this bugs me, not to conceptualize it adequately"
(079). After a short pause he started to consider the case where "the spring
to start with is not sprung at all. It's a—circle with a break in it" (079). He
drew a single coil with a break (figure 3.12) and stated "now that is your
paradigmatic spring—it doesn't even have any slope yet" (079).

Clement related to me that the videotape shows that S2 traced a circle
about seven inches in the air in front of himself as he stated "I'm just
trying to imagine the coil," (079) followed by a six-second pause prior to
drawing it. He then considered a force pushing it down while drawing

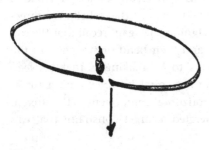

Figure 3.12
S2's single horizontal coil drawing.

the arrow. Here he began to focus on the actual geometry of the spring, reduced by limiting-case analysis to a single segment, and its three-dimensional configuration.

Note that S2 had previously drawn a single coil segment (figure 3.9) as we discussed in section 3.4.3. However, this figure is ambiguous in orientation and is not annotated with an arrow. One could consider it as either two-dimensional or three-dimensional, and he does not say which. The context of the drawing is the sheet with previous drawings of what he explicitly called two-dimensional figures (figure 3.6), so possibly that context also impeded his seeing immediately the implications of a three-dimensional representation of an open coil. Figure 3.12 was the first figure drawn on a new sheet, and when he would once again draw rods to examine again their slope, it was in the context of a quite different model of the stretch of a spring.

S2 considered once again winding the rod into a spring with circular coils and now inferred that the difference in slope arises because "somehow, when you wind it [the rod] up into a spring—it makes the varying slope go away. It's as though the varying slope is somehow geometrically converted—into—the 'coilingness' of the spring" (083).

Here S2 can be viewed as shifting back and forth between source constraints of rods and target constraints of springs by transforming the rod back into a wound-up spring. His focus now shifted to geometrical considerations by entertaining the possibility that "the cases [rod and spring] dynamically really are the same . . . but something purely geometrical is happening." Note that he now made several explicit references to the dynamics but continued to think that the problem lay in the geometrical differences and had "nothing to do with the dynamical forces involved." A lengthy segment of considering how a helix can be converted into a straight rod by cutting and opening it up in a cylindrical coordinate system followed this thought, leading to Model 5. In the midst of this reasoning he once again turned down an offer to end the session and go to lunch, saying, "grrr. . . . I'm—I'm finding it difficult to stop thinking about it" (103). The problem definitely had become his own!

Near the end of this segment, S2 fixed his attention on the drawing of the horizontal coil and while "visualizing this 8 [figure 3.13, number 8] being stretched again" (117), he drew a straight line (figure 3.13, number 9) and commented that the circle and the line are "paradigmatic" (117). That they are "paradigmatic" can be interpreted as S2's considering them as abstractions that capture what he takes to be salient about the cases of the wound-up spring and the unwound spring, respectively. However, drawing the line in the process of bending (figure 3.13, number 10) again

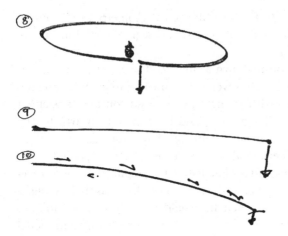

Figure 3.13
S2's drawings of rods in the context of the horizontal coil model.

revealed the increasing slope in the rod models, leading him back to the earlier inference that the rod and the spring coil seem not of the same type with respect to the mechanisms that cause the bending of the rod and the stretching of the spring.

At this point S2 expressed frustration that "I keep circling back to these same issues without getting anywhere with them," and the need to think about the problem in a "radically different way" (117). He decided to focus on the fact that the coils of a spring are circular, and whether there is anything about circularity that is significant to the slope. It is important to understand that his considerations of circularity are now in the significantly different context of constraint T10 that the coiling is in the horizontal plane. The open horizontal coil model, since it is situated in that plane with the stretch in the third, vertical, dimension, enables a different kind of mental simulation from the previous models. In figure 3.13, number 8, simulating a downward pull produces a vertical gap between corresponding points on a coiled wire. The downward pull in the horizontal plane, operating on the simplified geometry of a circle, opened the possibility of inferring a new mechanism of twisting in the stretch of a spring.

3.4.5   Model 5: Polygonal Coil
At this point S2 began to seek to reconcile the rod and horizontal coil models. He achieved this by integrating the derived target constraints of

lying in the horizontal plane and uniform distortion (T9–10) with the rod
model by creating a hybrid rod–spring model of a different kind with
respect to the mechanism of stretching from the earlier rod–spring models
(Models 2 and 3). Merging spring and rod constraints in the new context
led to his constructing a polygonal coil model—a horizontal coil made up
of rod segments—that enabled the key insight that there is twisting when
a spring stretches, and inferring that this is what accounts for the uniform
stretch of the spring.

The segment in which S2 constructed a series of polygonal coil models
began with his asking the questions:

What—what could the circularity do? Why should it matter? How would it change
the way the force is transmitted from increment to increment of the spring?
(117).

Notice that though still focused on the geometry, he was now explicitly
considering the force involved in stretching. S2 recognized that transmitting the force incrementally along the circle in the horizontal plane
stretches it bit by bit, as though it had joints, but with even distribution.
This inference was followed immediately by merging the models into a
hybrid rod–spring model—what I am calling a polygonal coil–model.

S2:   Aha! Now this is interesting. I—I imag—; I recalled my idea of the square spring
and—and the square is sort of like a circle, and I wonder what if I—what if I start
with a rod—and bend it once—and then I bend it again.—What if I produce a successive series of approximations to—(117)
Interviewer: hmm—
S2:   the circle, by producing a series of polygons! [. . .] That's constructing a continuous bridge [. . .] between the two cases. [. . .] clearly there can't be a hell of a
lot of difference between the circle and say a hexagon. (119)

In thinking about bending the rod in jointlike fashion, S2 appears to be
attempting to ascertain if a rod coiled up this way in the horizontal plane
and a circle stretching under a force transmitted incrementally are of the
same kind with respect to the mechanism of the stretch. At the end of this
section, S2 drew a hexagonal coil with a break in 3-D perspective (figure
3.14, number 11) and saw immediately that the hexagonal model is a
model of a different type from any he considered before for how the constraints would interact in the dynamic case.

We can interpret S2 here as reasoning that coils in the shape of polygons
can, in this context, be considered of the same kind, geometrically, as the
circular coil. That is, hexagons or squares can be taken to represent generic
polygons, and polygons approximate circles in the limit; that is, as one

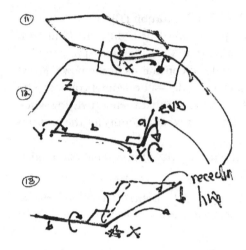

Figure 3.14
S2's drawing of the polygonal coils.

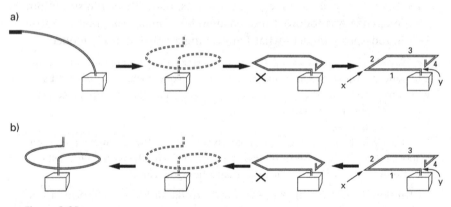

Figure 3.15
My rendering of S2's inferences based on generic models.

imagines the segments becoming infinitesimally small, as I have illustrated
in figure 3.15. Figure 3.15a represents sequences of inferences after he
inferred "a square is sort of like a circle" and considered bending the rod
up into various polygonal coils, and figure 3.15b represents the extrapolation to the limit, supporting his inference there is not a lot of "difference
between a circle and say a hexagon."

S2's next statement described a mental simulation that provided a crucial
insight:

Just looking at this it occurs to me that when force is applied here [he draws a downward pointing arrow at the end of the line segment], you not only get a bend on this segment, but because there's a pivot here [points to the "X" in figure 3.14, number 11], you get a torsion effect—around here [points to the adjacent segment]. (121)

That is, he inferred that there would be a twisting in the segments—producing a torsional strain in the wire—from mentally simulating the motion of the open segment of the horizontal coil in the dynamical case where the force from the weight operates on the coil oriented in the horizontal plane (as annotated with arrows in the drawing). He quite likely drew on his knowledge of physics at this point, in calling the twisting at the joint a "torsion effect." He went on:

Aha!—Maybe the behavior of the spring has something to do with the twist forces" [Clement 2005, 3, records that S2 moved his hands as if twisting an object, and continued to make either twisting or bending motions as the reasoning about the polygonal coil model unfolded.] That's a real interesting idea—That might be the key insight—that might be the key difference between this [flexible rod], which involves no torsion, and this [hexagonal coil]. (122)

As Clement characterized this aha! moment, here S2 has made "a major breakthrough in the solution," which can be viewed as a significant scientific insight because "by considering torsion the subject introduces a new causal factor into the system. Torsion constitutes a very different mechanism from bending for explaining how the spring resists stretching" (Clement 1988, 366). My interpretation adds that rotating the coil into the horizontal plane offers a three-dimensional perspective that affords a novel simulation that literally exhibits the twist, thus leading to his inference that for the spring the mechanism of stretch is torsion.

Moving on, S2 then constructed a square coil version of a polygonal coil model (figure 3.14, number 12) in order to accentuate the torsion effect, and he considered the possibility that torsion is what "stops the spring from—from flopping" (126). Exploring the properties of this model convinced him that unlike the initial rod model, this hybrid satisfies the uniform slope constraint T9. Both the hexagon and the square models incorporate features of the rod because straight line segments will bend. But the right angle of the square model means that both twisting and bending "start over again" (122) at each of the joints, rather than accumulating. Torsion does not accumulate, but

distributes itself equally across all the joints [. . .] so the twist doesn't get more [. . .] indeed we have a structure here which doesn't have this increasing slope at the bottom. (130)

Thus the square model captures the dynamical relational structure between the stretch of the spring and the deformation of the wire. When the model was constructed as lying in the horizontal plane, as with the polygonal coil (satisfying constraint T10), it afforded the possibility to imagine a twisting that is in the same relation to each piece so that the "springiness" is distributed evenly (satisfying constraint T9). Thus the polygonal coil models and the spring are of the same kind with respect to the torsion mechanism of stretch, or as S2 expressed it:

I feel I have a good model of sp—of a spring—Now I realize the reason a spring doesn't flop is because a lot of the springiness comes from torsion effects rather than from bendy effects. (132)

S2 went on to increase his confidence in his answer to the problem. If the width of a square coil is doubled, the increase in bending and torsion would also increase the stretch. The expression of increased confidence was then followed by a lengthy segment in which S2 explicitly explored how the torsion mechanism distributes the twist "as one approximates a circle more and more" (146). He drew the final figure (figure 3.14, number 13) to demonstrate to the interviewer what he meant by calling parts of the square model a fulcrum and a lever. I interpret S2 in the final analysis as working out how the twist force distributes in a spring by mentally extrapolating the polygonal coil models to the limit of a circular coil. What is left implicit in making the inference from the polygonal coil model to the spring is the earlier idea that squares and circles are not all that different. As we can see in figure 3.15b, extrapolating back from the square to the circle, the torsion in the spring would be evenly distributed and the bending effect disappears. That is, taking the square, the hexagon, and the polygonal figures "in the limit as one keeps making the segments smaller and the bend smaller . . . yeah and the angle of the bends is smaller" (162). From this it is clear that S2 understands that the torsion would spread out in such a way as to become a uniform property of the spring. He thus felt warranted in transferring the inference from the polygonal coil model to the spring.

Although S2's answer to the initial problem posed by Clement remains unchanged, that is, the spring with wider coils will stretch farther, S2's understanding of a spring is considerably altered. His initial concept of spring includes a vague notion that "springiness"—the stretch of a spring—is equated with bending. At the end of the problem-solving session, his concept of spring includes the notion that "springiness" involves twisting and that torsion can explain the uniform slope of a spring. He now knew, also, that dynamically rods and springs do not belong to the same class of phenomena with respect to the mechanisms of stretch. Once the session had ended, Clement explicitly questioned S2 as to whether he had been recently thinking about anything related to his reasoning or drawings. S2 asserted that he had not and that in fact the most he had ever done in a physics course was to think about elasticity, "the coefficient of $F = -kx$ or $F = kx$ or whatever [. . .] it can be anything elastic and the fact that it's coiled is irrelevant [. . .] we never talked about the different ways springiness came about, all we talked about was the formula, and its implications, and the way a spring behaved" (190). Knowing this equation, known as Hooke's law ($F = -kx$), would not have been helpful for answering the present spring problem because the problem is about the details of what might determine the spring constant k. It is possible that S2's physics knowledge might have provided him with the representation of the stretch of a spring as evenly distributed, but it did not provide him with the notion that torsion is the force that creates the even stretch. He derived this notion through the incremental modeling processes we have examined. At the end, S2 had constructed a novel concept of spring for himself, more in accord with the scientific representation, where torsion is the primary cause of deformation found in springs.

3.5   Discussion: S2's Model-based Reasoning Practices

As discussed earlier, my interest in the S2 protocol arose because of striking parallels between the ways S2 and Maxwell reasoned by constructing and manipulating models to solve problems leading to conceptual change. Thus, in the context of this book, I am presenting the S2 case as a parallel exemplar of such creative reasoning in science but "writ small." Whereas Maxwell added a new representational device to the conceptual and analytical resources of the physics community, S2 just provided one for himself. What the S2 case adds to my overall argument, however, is a detailed record of the visual and simulative dimensions of his reasoning processes in the course of problem solving, which we can only hypothesize from the records for the Maxwell case.

The S2 protocol gives more information on the modes of model-based reasoning used during the process than can historical records, which, of course, were created in different circumstances and for other purposes. We can, for instance, hypothesize that Maxwell could have recognized that the decrease in simulated velocity along the single vortex corresponded to the decrease in magnetic force along a Faradayan line of force if he had visualized this element of Model 1, the vortex medium, or that mentally simulating the motion of several vortices packed together in that medium could have led him to recognize the problem of jamming which led to Model 2, the vortex–idle wheel model, as a way of eliminating friction. In the case of S2, his utterances, drawings, and gestures while reasoning provide more direct evidence for visual and simulative components of model-based reasoning.

In what follows I summarize the major parallels between S2's and Maxwell's reasoning processes leading to their conceptual innovations. First, paralleling Maxwell's overall processes, S2's modeling processes, sche-matically represented in figure 3.16, consisted of integrating constraints drawn from the target domain of springs and analogical source domains

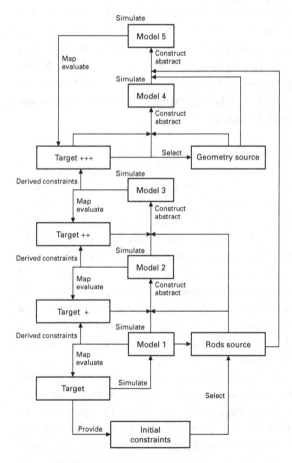

Figure 3.16
S2's modeling process.

of flexible rods and geometry into a series of models. Through these he attempted to construct a model that explains how a spring stretches. In both cases there was no ready-to-hand analogy from which to make mappings and draw inferences about the target problems. In the S2 exemplar, the domain of rods served as an initial source from which to derive constraints for constructing intermediary models. These are compared with the target spring to determine whether the mechanism of stretch is of the same kind as the mechanism of the stretch of a spring. In both cases the reasoner created models that are hybrid constructions of the targets and sources: S2's rod–spring models (the zigzag, rigid connector, and polygonal coil models) and Maxwell's vortex–idle wheel models. These physically implausible models were productive for reasoning because many aspects that would be required of a fully working physical entity were left unspecified (see the discussion below on generic modeling).

Second, throughout the modeling process S2 went through cycles in which he critically evaluated the plausibility of the models and the inferences he drew from them, and made adaptations in light of insights and newly derived constraints (as Clement has also argued). This is strikingly similar to the cycles of Maxwell's model criticism and revision, although it happens on a different time scale since Maxwell's problem was much more difficult.

Third, the protocol provides strong evidence that S2 reasoned through imagistic model construction, manipulation, and simulation. Although S2 did not state that he mentally simulated the spring as unwinding in creating Model 1, the fact that he continually referred to the rod as the "unwound spring" supports my interpretation. Next, the visually evident nonconstant slope of the imagined bending rod cued S2's inference that the stretched spring has a constant slope and that the rod does not. To assure himself of this he drew rods and springs in order to "fix [them] visually." He called the nature of his imagistic simulations of the motions "kinesthetic," indicating he was attempting to draw on sensorimotor experiences and related these to how springs and rods move. Indeed, he often accompanied visualization attempts with gestures, such as a twisting motion when simulating bending in the segments of the hexagonal coil model, which led him to recognize that there is a twisting force on a stretching spring. Throughout the protocol, S2 spoke of visualizing models, drew several schematic representations, and used gestures while simulating dynamical processes to be performed with the models and to provide a three-dimensional perspective. Further, we can make explicit links between specific drawings S2 produced and his verbalizations about visualizing or imagining what he is representing. This kind of information adds plausibility to my hypothesis that Maxwell's drawings and descriptive texts of simulations were also accompanied by mental visualizations and simulations.

Fourth, S2 used various forms of abstractive reasoning including idealization, limits, and generic modeling. In particular, the process I have called "abstraction via generic modeling" (see section 2.3.2), which we saw played a significant role in Maxwell's modeling, is also significant in S2's reasoning. For instance, S2's inferences apply to springs in general, such as that a spring of any size and shape would have constant slope on stretching under a weight. Most importantly, this form of abstraction figures in making the topological transformations and justifying the inferences S2 made from them. Problems that arose in simulating the stretching of the zigzag and rigid connector models, which are concatenations of rods, directed him to focus on the circular nature of spring coils, to draw on the source domain of geometrical figures, and, ultimately, to construct generic topological transformations of these hybrid rod–spring models, which I illustrate in figure 3.17.

S2 was led to consider topological transformations once he had drawn the spring coil as a "circle with a break in it," which centered his attention on the coil as lying in the horizontal plane. The topological transformations, circle to hexagon and hexagon to square, created a hybrid model—a generic polygonal coil—in which he could examine the behaviors of

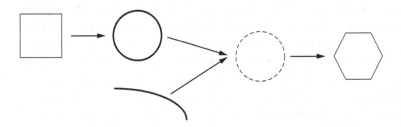

"Aha! Now this is interesting. I -- I imag --; I recalled my idea of the square spring and... and the square is sort of like a circle, and I wonder what if I... what if I star with a rod... and bend it once... and then I bend it again... What if I produce a successive series of approximations to ---- "

"the circle, by producing a series of polygons! [......] That's constructing a continuous bridge [......] between the two cases. [......] clearly there can't be a hell of a lot of difference between the circle and say a hexagon." (117–119)

Figure 3.17
Example of S2's generic topological transformations.

As recognized through the behavior of constructed hexagonal model

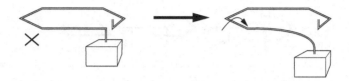

As exaggerated through the behavior of constructed square model

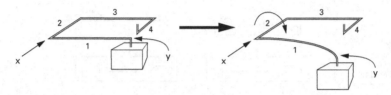

As force is applied at y not only does rod 1 bend, rod 2 twists

Figure 3.18
S2's discovery of torsion.

both the rod and spring together, and this led to the key insight: the "aha!" moment of the inference that torsion is what keeps the spring "from flopping," as I have illustrated in figure 3.18.

The transformation from the hexagon, where torsion was recognized, to a square exaggerated—and more clearly separated—twist from bend. Once torsion was recognized, the twist was imaginatively distributed along the coil of a spring by imagining the rod segments getting "smaller and smaller," thus keeping the slope constant when it is stretched (see figure 3.19).

I have called Model 5 a model of a *generic* polygonal coil because the way S2 reasons, any finite-sided polygon that could be drawn could be substituted for it. This can be seen, for example, in his assertions that there are no salient differences in this context between a polygonal coil and a circular one, so inferences derived from polygonal coils should apply to circular coils. That is, in the context of considering the dynamical behavior of a coiled spring, circles can be considered as belonging to the class of polygonal figures. Figure 3.19 demonstrates the legitimacy of transferring the inference that torsion is distributed evenly in the stretching of a spring through reasoning that extrapolates the segments from a definite size to smaller and smaller segments.

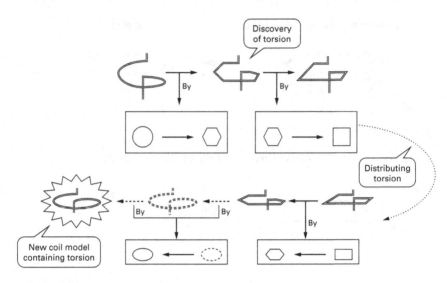

Figure 3.19
Sequence of generic transformation in discovering torsion.

There are obvious places where the modeling processes of Maxwell and S2 differ, but none that makes any difference for using either as an exemplar of model-based reasoning in conceptual change. One significant difference is that unlike Maxwell, S2 did not derive equations. When questioned at the completion of the problem-solving process, he did have a vague recollection of a mathematical representation for elastic objects, but this equation does not provide an understanding of the mechanism of stretch. Knowing just the equation would have left him in much the same situation as Maxwell's bellringer—with no understanding of the underlying mechanism—but S2's problem required understanding the mechanism in order to solve it satisfactorily. This aspect resulted in his conceptual innovation.

As in the Maxwell case, the answer to the puzzle of how S2 was able to create a fundamentally novel representation for himself—one in which the stretch of a spring is governed by torsion—lies in seeing that S2 reasoned through constructing intermediary, hybrid models that embodied constraints from both rod sources and the spring target. In particular, the abstractive processes of generic modeling, which mainly involved generic topological transformations, enabled S2 to integrate rod and spring constraints into the horizontal coil model from which a fundamentally new (to him) representational structure emerged—one that exhibited the mechanism of torsion.

4   The Cognitive Basis of Model-based Reasoning Practices: Mental Modeling

The proposition is a model of reality as we imagine it.

—Ludwig Wittgenstein, *Tractatus Logico-Philosophicus*

vdH: You seem to visualize all these problems?

Tao: [N]owadays to solve a problem it's not enough to write down all sorts of formulas: you have to form some kind of a mental model. You have to get some rough picture and work on that first. And that's how everybody is working now is my experience. That's the hard part.

vdH: To get a grip on the idea behind the formulas?

Tao: Yes, there is the story that Richard Feynman, the famous physicist . . . One day his wife caught him when he was just rolling around with his eyes closed. And she was very worried and said: Richard what are you doing? And he said: I'm trying to see what it feels like being an electron. Actually I have done something very similar when I was a child. My Dad caught me when I was just tilting back and forth trying to feel what it was to be a wave—I didn't realize my dad was watching me.

—Terrance Tao, NRC Handelsblad interview with Margriet van der Heijden, April 21, 2007[1]

In this chapter, I address the problem of the nature of the cognitive representations and processing that could underlie the kind of model-based reasoning in which scientists engage during conceptual innovation and other problem solving. I argue that the cognitive basis for the model-based reasoning practices exhibited in the exemplars, and employed widely and variously by scientists, lies in the human capacity for simulative thinking through mental modeling. This capacity is rooted in the ability to imagine—to depict in the mind—both real-world and imaginary situations, and to make inferences about future states of these situations based on current understandings, with and in the absence of physical instantiations of the things being reasoned about. My analysis brings together several strands of research in cognitive science to develop an account of mental modeling sufficient for model-based reasoning in science.

Thinking about the scientific domain has required extending the investigation beyond the literatures specifically on mental models to include research on imaginative simulation in mental imagery, mental animation, and perception-based representation. Further, within traditional cognitive science, the representations and processing involved in reasoning are held to be located "in the head," and reasoning is analyzed as detached from the material environments in which it occurs. Although it is possible that simple model-based reasoning could take place only "in the head," reasoning of the complexity of that in science makes extensive use of external representations. A wide range of data—historical, protocol, and ethnographic—establishes that many kinds of external representations are used during scientific reasoning: linguistic (descriptions, narratives, written and verbal communications), mathematical equations, visual representations, gestures, physical models, and computational models. Thus even an analysis of *mental* modeling needs to consider the relations among the internal and external representations and processes in problem solving. I conclude with considering the question of the nature of the mental representations used in mental modeling such as to enable the internal and external representational coupling during reasoning processes. Taken together, the literatures make a compelling case for simulative model-based reasoning and representational coupling.

4.1   The Mental Models Framework

The notion of a "mental model" is central to much of contemporary cognitive science. In 1943, the psychologist and physiologist Kenneth Craik hypothesized that in many instances people reason by carrying out thought experiments on internal models of physical situations, where a model is a structural, behavioral, or functional analogue to a real-world phenomenon (Craik 1943). Craik based his hypothesis on the predictive power of thought and the ability of humans to explore real-world and imaginary situations mentally. We will return to Craik's view in a later section, after first considering its contemporary legacy. Craik made this proposal at the height of the behaviorist approach in psychology, and so it received little notice. The development of a "cognitive" psychology in the 1960s created a more hospitable environment for investigating and articulating the hypothesis. A new edition of Craik's book with a postscript replying to critics in 1967 fell on more fertile ground and has since had considerable impact on contemporary cognitive science. Since the early 1980s, a "mental models framework" has developed in a large segment of cognitive science. This explanatory framework posits models as organized units of mental representation of knowledge that are employed in various cognitive tasks, including reasoning, problem solving, and discourse comprehension.

What is a "mental model"? How is it represented? What kinds of processing underlie its use? What are the mental mechanisms that create and use mental models? How does mental modeling engage external representations and processes? These issues are not often addressed explicitly in the literature, and where they are, there is as yet no consensus that might serve as a theory of mental models. Thus, I have chosen the word "framework" to characterize a wide range of research. What the positions within this framework share is a general hypothesis that some mental representations of domain knowledge are organized in units containing knowledge of spatiotemporal structure, causal connections, and other relational structures.

Having wrestled with a considerable portion of the cognitive science literature on mental models, I have to concur with Lance Rips's observation that much use of the notion appears "muddled" (Rips 1986), but I disagree with his conclusion that dismisses the viability of the notion entirely. A potentially quite powerful notion can be articulated and, as some researchers have contended, could provide a much-needed unifying framework for the study of cognition (see, e.g., Gilhooly 1986; Johnson-Laird 1980). My objective here is modest: to provide a clarification of the idea of reasoning through mental modeling, an integrative analysis that is consistent with the cognitive science research on mundane cases and is adequate as a cognitive basis for the scientific model-based reasoning practices, which can then be investigated further in empirical and theoretical research in cognitive science. As noted previously, there are no cognitive theories sitting on the shelf, ready to use in "explaining" science. Thus, this analysis meets an objective of the cognitive-historical method, which is to inject considerations from the cognitive practices of scientists into the analyses of cognition in general.

A "mental model" is a structural, behavioral, or functional analog representation of a real-world or imaginary situation, event, or process. It is analog in that it preserves constraints inherent in what is represented. In the early 1980s, several largely independent strands of research emerged introducing the theoretical notions of "mental model" and "mental modeling" into the cognitive science literature. One strand introduced the notion to explain the effects of semantic information in logical reasoning (Johnson-Laird 1983). Another strand introduced the notion to explain the empirical finding that in reasoning related to discourse comprehension, people seem to reason from a representation of the structure of a situation rather than from a description of a situation (so-called "discourse" and "situation" models, Johnson-Laird 1982; Perrig and Kintsch 1985). Both of these strands focused on the nature of the representations constructed in working memory during reasoning and problem-solving tasks. Yet another strand introduced the notion in relation to long-term memory representations of knowledge used in understanding and reasoning, in particular about physical systems. This literature posited the notion to explain a wide range of experimental results indicating that people use organized knowledge structures relating to physical systems in attempting to understand manual control systems and devices in the area of human–machine interaction (see Rouse and Morris 1986 for an overview) and in employing qualitative domain knowledge of physical systems to solve problems (Gentner and Stevens 1983). Some of the early work relating to physical systems that began with psychological studies migrated into AI where computational theories of "naive" or "qualitative" physics in particular were developed to explore issues of knowledge organization, use, access, and control, such as in understanding and predicting the behavior of liquids (Hayes 1979) or the motion of a ball in space and time (Forbus 1983). Much of the pioneering research in the third strand is represented in the edited collection *Mental Models* (Gentner and Stevens 1983), which appeared the same year as Johnson-Laird's (1983) monograph of the same name that brought together the strands on working memory.

Research within the mental models framework is so extensive and varied that an inventory is not possible. As an indication of the range, examples of research include: AI models of qualitative reasoning about causality in physical systems (Bobrow 1985), representations of intuitive domain knowledge in various areas, such as physics and astronomy (Vosniadou and Brewer 1992), analogical problem solving (Gentner and Stevens 1983), deductive and inductive reasoning (Holland et al. 1986; Johnson-Laird and Byrne 1993), probabilistic inference (Kahneman and Tversky 1982), "heterogeneous" or "multimodal" reasoning (Allwein and Barwise 1996), modal logic (Bell and Johnson-Laird 1998), narrative and discourse comprehension (Johnson-Laird 1982; Perrig and Kintsch 1985), scientific thought experiments (Nersessian 1991, 1992), and cultural transmission (Shore 1997). However, a consensus view has not developed among these areas of research. The preponderance of research into mental models has been involved with specifying the content and structure of long-term memory models in a specific domain or with respect to specific reasoning tasks or

levels of expertise, and not with addressing the more foundational questions raised above. Most importantly, clarification is needed on basic issues
as to the nature of the format of the model and the processing involved
in using a model.

Given that my focus is on mental modeling during reasoning processes,
I consider here only the psychological accounts that hypothesize reasoning
as involving the construction and manipulation of a model in working
memory during the reasoning process and not the accounts of the nature
of representation in long-term memory, about which my account can
remain agnostic. Of course reasoning processes draw on long-term memory
representations, and so an account of these processes can lead to insights
into the nature of the stored representations that support reasoning and
understanding. Additionally, in conceptual change, the expectation is that
changes arrived at through reasoning would lead to changes in the content
and structure of long-term memory representations. I also will not address
accounts that are primarily computational since what Rips (1986) pointed
out still holds today: computational modeling of qualitative reasoning
requires highly complex representations that in the end can only do much
simpler reasoning than humans can carry out. He considered this a reason
for dismissing the very notion of mental modeling, whereas I would counter
that the limitations of the computational models stem from the nature of
representations and processing made use of so far, and that these quite
possibly do not adequately capture the human cognitive phenomena.

Working memory accounts of mental modeling include those concerned
with reasoning and with narrative and discourse comprehension. The
literatures on imaginative simulation in mental imagery, mental animation, perception-based representation, and ideomotor theory also provide
insights relevant to developing an account of mental modeling. My strategy is first to address some general issues about representation and processing that we will need in discussing mental modeling, next to briefly survey
the accounts in the literatures, then to propose a synthesis of the several
threads in the research to address simulative model-based reasoning as
practiced by scientists, and finally to return to the implications of all this
for conceptual change.

4.2 General Format and Processing Issues

It has been a fundamental presupposition of cognitive science that humans
think about real and imaginary worlds through internal symbolic representations. Although that assumption has been challenged by researchers

in the areas of connectionism, dynamic cognition, and situated cognition, in this section I focus on the controversy about the nature of mental representation as it appears within traditional cognitive science, where there are mental representations and "internal" and "external" are clear and distinct notions. Later in the chapter I argue for the position that internal and external representations used in reasoning processes form a coupled system.

The founding assumptions were reiterated and elaborated upon by Alonso Vera and Herbert Simon (Vera and Simon 1993) in response to criticisms. They specify a "physical symbol system" as possessing a memory capable of storing symbols and symbol structures and a set of information processes that form symbols and structures as a function of stimuli, which in humans are sensory stimuli. Sensory stimuli produce symbol structures that cause motor actions, which in turn modify symbol structures in memory. Such a physical symbol system interacts with the environment by receiving sensory information from it and converting these into symbol structures in memory and by acting upon it in ways determined by those symbol structures. Perceptual and motor processes connect symbol structures with the environment, thus providing a semantics for the symbols. In the case of humans, then, all representation and processing is internal to the human mind–brain.

What is the nature of the symbols and the symbol structures? Since its inception, there has been a deep divide in the field of cognitive science between those who hold that all mental representation is language-like and those who hold that at least some representation is perceptual or imagistic in format. Herbert Simon reports that this divide "nearly torpedoed the effort of the Sloan Foundation to launch a major program of support for cognitive science" (Simon 1977, 385). Volumes of research have since been directed toward and against each side of the divide, and even with significant clarification of the issues and considerable experimental work, the problem remains unresolved and most likely will continue to be until more is known about the nature of the representation-creating mechanisms in the brain. The format issue is important because different kinds of representation—linguistic, formulaic, imagistic, analog—enable different kinds of processing operations. In what follows I distinguish aspects or components of representations as "propositional," "iconic," "amodal," and "modal." A representation of a state of affairs can be composed of combinations of these, and thus be "heterogeneous" or "multimodal" (see, e.g., Glashow, Chandrasekharan, and Narayanan 1995), such as a diagram annotated with language.

Operations on linguistic and formulaic representations include the familiar operations of logic and mathematics. Linguistic representations, for example, are interpreted as referring to physical objects, structures, processes, or events descriptively. Customarily, the relationship between this kind of representation and the interpretation of what it refers to is "truth," and thus the representation is evaluated as being true or false. Constructing these representations requires following a grammar that specifies the proper syntactical structures. Operations on such representations are rule-based and truth-preserving if the symbols are interpreted in a consistent manner and the properties they refer to are stable in that environment. Additional operations can be defined in limited domains provided they are consistent with the constraints that hold in that domain. Manipulation of a linguistic or formulaic representation of a model would require explicit representation of salient parameters, including constraints and transition states. Condition–action rules of production systems provide an example, as do the equation-like representations of qualitative process models. This latter case allows for simulative reasoning about physical systems through changing the values of variables to create new states of the model. I will call the aspects of representations with these characteristics "propositional," following the usual philosophical usage that refers to a language-like encoding possessing a vocabulary, grammar, and semantics (see, e.g., Fodor 1975) rather than the usage sometimes employed in cognitive science, as coextensive with "symbolic."

On the other hand, analog models, diagrams, and imagistic representations are interpreted as representing demonstratively. The relationship between this kind of representation, which I will call "iconic," and what it represents is similarity or goodness of fit (with isomorphism being the limit).[2] Iconic representations are interpreted as being similar, in degrees and aspects, to what they represent, and are thus evaluated as using notions such as "accurate" or "inaccurate." Operations on iconic representations involve transformations of the representations that change their properties and relations in ways consistent with the constraints of the domain. Significantly, transformational constraints pertaining to iconic representations can be implicit. For example, a person can do simple reasoning about what happens when a rod is bent without having an explicit rule, such as "given the same force a longer rod will bend farther." The form of representation is such as to enable simulations in which the model behaves in accord with constraints that need not be stated explicitly during this process. Mathematical expressions present an interesting case in that it is conceivable they can be represented mentally either propositionally or iconically (see, e.g., Kurz and Tweney 1998). Although their written appearance is in language-like format, it is conceivable that in some reasoning tasks the mental representation of, for example, a curl (∇x) or a divergence ($\nabla\bullet$), would be iconic in nature.

Dispersed throughout the cognitive science literature is another distinction pertinent to the format of mental models, which concerns the nature of the symbols that constitute propositional and iconic representations—that between "amodal" and "modal" symbols (see, e.g., Barsalou 1999). Modal symbols are analog representations of the perceptual states from which they are extracted. Amodal symbols are arbitrary transductions from perceptual states, such as those associated with a "language of thought." A modal symbol representing a cat, for instance, would retain perceptual aspects of cats, such as a general outline of shape; an amodal symbol would have an arbitrary relationship to the cat such as the way that the strings of letters of the words "cat" or "chat" or "Katz" are arbitrarily related to the perceptual aspects of cats. Propositional representations, in the sense discussed above, are composed of amodal symbols. Iconic representations can be composed of either, including combinations. For example, a representation of the situation "the circle is to the left of the square, which is to the left of the triangle" could be composed of either modal tokens, such as ●—■—▲, or amodal tokens, standing for these entities in much the way the words "circle," "square," and "triangle" correspond to objects (in this configuration, the representation of the relation "to the left of" is modal). Whether the mental symbols used in an iconic representation are modal or amodal has implications for how such representations are constructed and manipulated. Constructing a modal representation, for example, potentially involves a reactivation of patterns of neural activity in the perceptual and motor areas of the brain that were activated in the initial experience of something. Thus, manipulation of the representation is likely to involve perceptual and motor processing, whereas an amodal representation is typically held not to involve such processing.

One difficulty in sorting through the mental modeling literature is that one can find all possible flavors in it, which, for brevity, I characterize as propositional, amodal iconic, and modal iconic mental models. Among those giving working memory accounts, Holland et al. (1986) maintain that reasoning with a mental model is a process of applying condition-action rules to propositional representations of the specific situation. For instance, making inferences about a feminist bank teller, "Jane," would involve constructing a model from various amodal symbols referring to feminists and bank tellers. On Johnson-Laird's account, mental models are not propositional; rather they are iconic with amodal symbols as constituents. Making a logical inference such as modus ponens occurs by manipulating amodal tokens in a spatial array that captures the salient structural dimensions of the problem and then searching for counterexamples to the model transformation. "Depictive mental models" (Schwartz and Black 1996a) provide an example of modal iconic mental models. Making an inference through a depictive model involves manipulating modal symbols, such as of the components of a schematic model of a setup of machine gears in the configuration of interest, using tacit knowledge embedded in constraints to simulate possible behaviors. The modal representation of the gears facilitates the reasoner's use of tacit knowledge without it having to be explicit. In both instances of iconic models, operations on a mental model transform it in ways consistent with the constraints of the system it represents.

Although the jury is still out on the format issues of working memory representations, the research that investigates reasoning about physical systems leads in the iconic direction, which, as I will discuss below, was the initial proposal by Craik. The issues of the nature of long-term memory representations and the working memory format and processes involved in reasoning will need eventually to be resolved in the mental models framework. However, making progress on understanding model-based reasoning in science does not require these issues to be settled. My analysis of model-based reasoning need only adopt a minimalist hypothesis: in certain problem-solving tasks, humans reason by constructing and manipulating an iconic mental model of the situations, events, and processes in working memory. The hypothesis leaves open, however, the questions of the nature of the representations in long-term memory, and whether the working memory representation employed in reasoning has amodal or modal constituents. In section 4.4.5, I will make the stronger hypothesis that these representations do have modal aspects.

One final general issue needs discussion: Are iconic aspects of representations reducible to propositional ones, thus rendering issues of difference in format and processing moot? Two distinctions made by Larkin and Simon (1987) concerning diagrams and propositions transfer to this case. The first is the distinction between *levels of implementation* and *levels of structures and processes,* and the second is the distinction between *informational* and *computational equivalence.* With respect to the first distinction, what they argue is that although it is possible that at the level of implementation in the brain or in the hardware of a computer all representation is the same, this does not entail that representation at the higher level of structures and processes is the same as that employed at the implementation level. The human brain, for example, could be the type of computational system that employs propositional representations at the level of implementation and iconic representations in many of its higher-level processes. Their formulation, however, assumes independence of the two levels. This assumption holds for computers, but might not for humans and other biological systems. The functioning of many kinds of systems depends on what they are implemented in, and not enough is known about the brain to judge in advance whether or not it is this kind of system. It is an open and empirical problem in need of investigation in the neurosciences—not something that can be stipulated a priori.

Still, their point that different kinds of representations could be easier to use for specific situations or purposes is useful. For example, humans and other biological species could have greater facility in, and ease of, problem solving through manipulating iconic representations, even though for a similar task a digital computer would use only propositional representations. In considering this possibility, Simon and Larkin were led to introduce the second distinction, that between *informationally equivalent* and *computationally equivalent* representations. Forms of representation are informationally equivalent if they can be translated into one another without loss of content. The weak claim for iconic representation is that iconic representations are informationally equivalent to the corresponding propositional ones. The strong claim is that iconic representations contain information unavailable in propositional ones. Forms of representation are computationally equivalent if the nature of the processing is the same. The weak claim in support of iconic representations is that they make certain kinds of inferences easier for humans. The strong claim is that certain kinds of inferences are impossible without them. Even if both weak claims are the best that can be established, this leaves open the possibility that iconic representation play a significant role in human reasoning. Larkin and Simon (1987) make both weak claims, while arguing also that mental imagery likely plays a role in some human problem-solving tasks. They maintain that the argument has largely been engaged on the wrong side of the distinction, the informational side rather than the computational side. However, even if the issues were to be engaged on the computational side, only a *null* result for computational equivalence would support the position of strong propositionalists that all representation is amodal, and how this might be determined experimentally seems an intractable problem.

4.3 Mental Modeling in Logical Reasoning

Among the working memory accounts of mental modeling in reasoning, the *locus classicus* is the account of Philip Johnson-Laird's 1983 book *Mental Models*. Although Johnson-Laird intends the theoretical apparatus to extend to all kinds of reasoning, his own numerous investigations (see, e.g., 1984, 1990, 1995) and those of his coresearchers, most notably Ruth Byrne (Johnson-Laird and Byrne 1991), have centered largely on logical reasoning. The original monograph derives from research both on logical reasoning and on discourse comprehension. Johnson-Laird first tested the mental modeling hypothesis in the paradigmatic domain of deductive inference, where, on the traditional view, it seems unquestionable that formal rules of inference are applied to propositional representations. In contrast, he argued that much research on untutored logical competence demonstrates that humans can reason validly without needing "recourse to mental logics with formal rules of inference" (1983, 41). There have been many other contributions to the mental modeling literature on logical reasoning, but since this is not intended as a survey, I focus on the highly influential early work of Johnson-Laird. I pass over much of what Johnson-Laird presents as the "theory" of mental models in order to keep the focus on issues pertaining to model-based reasoning practices. Johnson-Laird distinguishes three types of mental representation: *propositions*, "strings of symbols that correspond to natural language"; *mental models*, "structural analogues of the world"; and *images*, "perceptual correlates of models from a particular point of view" (1983, 165). In later work he reduced these types to two, since images are a "special sort of model—a two-dimensional representation that is projected from a three-dimensional model" (1989, 491).

Johnson-Laird's research on logical reasoning constitutes a response to an ongoing controversy in cognitive psychology about the nature of human reasoning that parallels the issues outlined in chapter 1 for philosophy. The development of symbolic logic in the late nineteenth and early twentieth centuries facilitated the traditional view of reasoning both in philosophy and in psychology. In psychology, too, language has long been held to be the way to illuminate mental faculties, and thus what can be done with language has dominated views of reasoning. On the traditional psychological view, the mental operations underlying reasoning consist in applying a mental logic to proposition-like representations. As expressed in the classic work by Jean Piaget and Barbel Inhelder, "reasoning is nothing more than the propositional calculus itself" (Inhelder and Piaget 1958). One reason for the development of the notion of mental modeling is that critics of the traditional view contend that a syntactical account of reasoning cannot account for the empirical evidence that semantic information plays a significant role even in logical reasoning. It also cannot account for the logical competence and systematic errors displayed by people with no training in logic. Unlike reasoning with formal logics, most human reasoning and problem solving *are* content- and context-dependent.

The Wason card task (Wason 1960; see Johnson-Laird 1983 for a discussion of it and subsequent research) is an early and now classic experiment that has had considerable impact in this field. In the task, the subject is presented with four cards, two displaying a letter (one consonant and one vowel) and two displaying a number (one even and one odd). Such a sequence might be: A G 2 5. The participant is told that each card has a number on one side and a letter on the other. The task is to determine how many cards have to be turned over in order to make a given generalization true, for instance, "if a card has a vowel on one side then it has an even number on the other side." Most participants fail to make the correct inference that both the A and the 5 cards need to be turned over. However, when meaningful information and relations are provided on the cards, the number of correct inferences increases dramatically. For example, simply substituting destinations and modes of transportation, such as "every time I go to Manchester, I travel by train" (Wason and Shapiro 1971) or postage stamp costs and sealed or unsealed envelopes for the letters and numbers (Johnson-Laird, Legrenzi, and Legrenzi 1972), increases the ability of subjects to reason correctly. The most significant increases occur with deontic conditions, such as "if a person is drinking beer, they must be over 21" (Griggs and Cox 1993).

Johnson-Laird (1983) claims his account of mental models originates in Craik's intuitive notion of a "relation-structure":

By a model we thus mean any physical or chemical system which has a similar relation-structure to that of the process it imitates. By "relation-structure" I do not mean some obscure non-physical entity which attends the model, but the fact that it is a physical working model which works in the same way as the process it parallels, in the aspects under consideration at any moment. Thus, the model need not resemble the real object pictorially; Kelvin's tide-predictor, which consists of a number of pulleys on levers, does not resemble a tide in appearance, but it works in the same way in certain essential respects. (Craik 1943, 51–52)

As I will discuss later, Johnson-Laird's emphasis on logical reasoning differs from Craik's, which was more concerned with simulative physical reasoning. On Johnson-Laird's account, a mental model is a structural analogue of a real-world or imaginary situation, event, or process that the mind constructs during reasoning. A mental model is a structural analogue in that it embodies a representation of the salient spatial and temporal relations among, and the causal structures connecting, the events and entities depicted and whatever other information that is relevant to the problem-solving task. Although he does not discuss this explicitly, as with Craik's view, the theory needs to include that mental models can also be behavioral and functional analogues. Johnson-Laird posits that in the case of language, information provided by a linguistic expression is first represented propositionally, and then "the semantics of the mental language maps propositional representations to mental models of real or imaginary worlds: *propositional representations are interpreted with respect to mental models*" (1983, 156, emphasis in the original). Information provided by perception is represented directly by a mental model, without the need of a propositional intermediary. He notes that although it is not yet known how the machinery of the brain constructs models, how it does so is a tractable problem, as in the case of vision where the mechanisms have largely been worked out.

Johnson-Laird is not explicit about the format of a mental model, but clearly wishes to distinguish it from a propositional representation. Unlike propositional representations, the structure of a mental model is analogous to the state of affairs described in a proposition or depicted in perception. Equally, he wishes to distinguish a mental model from the "picture in the mind" view he associates with some mental imagery claims. What evidence he provides supports the attribution that in format, he views a mental model as iconic. In most cases the model is highly schematic and composed of amodal symbols, where abstract relations are also represented amodally. That is, specific individuals and entities, such as "John is a beekeeper and Janet is an artist," are represented by different but arbitrary tokens. Generalizations, such as "All artists are beekeepers," which are represented by variables in formal logic, are represented in mental models by amodal tokens understood as representing the set of individuals or entities. A mental model is specific in that it is "a single representative from the set of models satisfying an assertion" (Johnson-Laird 1983, 264), but the interpretive processes are such that the model is treated as a "representative sample from a larger set" (ibid., 158), with conclusions attaining appropriate generality.

Simple examples of mental models are provided by the possible representations of the expression "it is raining or it is snowing":

a

    b

where the diagonal relation is interpreted to represent "or," and of the expression "it is raining and it is snowing":

a b

where the relation of being adjacent to is interpreted to represent "and." More complex relations can also be represented, such as "all artists are beekeepers," which can be represented as:

$a_1 = b$
$a_2 = b$

.

.

where "=" is interpreted to represent the identification of artists as beekeepers; and "Phil sold his car to George for \$100," which can be represented as:

Phil $\rightarrow$ car   George $\rightarrow$ \$100
Phil $\rightarrow$ \$100 George $\rightarrow$ car

where "$\rightarrow$" is interpreted to represent the ownership relation. That I use linguistic symbols should not be taken to indicate that the representations are propositional. One could equally as well use arbitrary symbols other than linguistic to represent Phil, George, and the car, as long as one is consistent.

Rather than employing rules of inference, the reasoner manipulates models to produce inferences in ways controlled by the operators associated with them. Many of these operations are of a spatial nature, such as those enabling the movement of tokens left, right, up, down, in front, in back, and so forth. Such operations would seem to involve perceptual mechanisms even if the tokens are amodal. Evaluation of an inference requires attempting to construct an alternative model. In the case of deductive logic, evaluation of inferences for validity consists of trying to devise models that instantiate counterexamples. Johnson-Laird argues that the need to search for alternatives requires an independent propositional representation of information provided in that format (1983, 165), so it can be used to attempt alternative constructions.

His claim that images are projections from models is problematic on an amodal interpretation, however, in that it would not account for the vivid imagery that some people experience. If the tokens are amodal then an image projected from a model could only be an abstract image arbitrarily related to its real-world correlate. In the few specific examples he provides of spatiotemporal relations and simulative reasoning, Johnson-Laird seems to entertain the possibility of modal representation for some aspects of the model. Examples he provides involving spatial relations support this interpretation, such as figuring one's way through a maze and "the fork is to the left (or picked up before, etc.) of the knife, which is to the left of the spoon," where the spatial relation "to the left" is represented modally even though the actual objects are represented with amodal tokens:

f k s

He allows that the model representation can range from a simple spatial arrangement to a three-dimensional spatiotemporal dynamic simulation of events and processes. However, it is unclear how, for example, causal information would be represented in the mental models such that inferences could be made directly through simulation of the state of affairs as represented.

Since my concern is not with logical reasoning per se, I will not go into the advantages and criticisms of his account of logical reasoning. In short, this line of research provides substantial evidence that, even in instances of classical logical inference, intuitive human reasoning often proceeds through creating and manipulating iconic mental models. As noted, what is not yet clear is how mental modeling can be used in reasoning that involves simulating physical processes. Here the literature on discourse and situation models, to which Johnson-Laird has also contributed, offers insight.[3]

4.4 "Craikian" Mental Modeling: Simulative Reasoning

Although Johnson-Laird roots his view in the earlier proposal of Craik, his focus on mental modeling in the domains of deductive, inductive, and modal reasoning tasks and his desire to distinguish mental models from what is customarily understood as mental imagery have led him to underplay or not develop what I take to be Craik's central insight: reasoning via mental simulation. Accounting for simulative reasoning about physical systems, and model-based reasoning in science in particular, requires more kinds of model manipulation than moving tokens in spatiotemporal configurations. Tacit and explicit domain knowledge of entities, behaviors, and processes, especially causal knowledge, is needed in constructing models and creating new states via simulation. For an intuitive understanding of what it means to mentally simulate, take the familiar situation where a large sofa needs to be moved through a doorway. The default approach to solving the problem is to imagine or mentally enact moving a mental token approximating the shape of the sofa through various rotations constrained by the boundaries of a doorway-like shape. We do not customarily resort to formulating a series of propositions and applying logic, or to doing trigonometric calculations. Situation-specific behavioral and causal knowledge (which need not be explicit) of characteristics about sofas and doorways come into play, for example, that standard sofas have little flexibility in bending or twisting, and that a doorframe will not usually give way when pressed upon by a sofa. Note also that arriving at a problem solution is easier if it is taking place in front of the doorway and the sofa, as opposed to in a furniture store when considering whether it is wise to purchase the sofa.

Clearly, in the case of science, the knowledge required to carry out such a simulation is more complex, but it is this primitive ability that underlies the more sophisticated mental modeling simulations performed by scientists. There are numerous reports by scientists and engineers of conducting mental transformations and simulations in solving problems. There is Kekule's claim to have imagined a snake biting its tale, and Einstein's claim to have imagined chasing a beam of light. Eugene Ferguson's fascinating analysis of the role of visual thinking in engineering practices in *Engineering and the Mind's Eye* (1992) provides many examples, most notably Nikola Tesla's report that part of his process of designing devices was to imagine the devices and run them in his imagination over a period of weeks in order to see which parts were most subject to wear. Although most expert accounts are anecdotal, as we will see, there is ample experimental evidence in cognitive science in support of reasoning through simulation in mundane and expert cases.

There are four points to highlight from mundane usage that will recur throughout the rest of this chapter and carry across in considering scientific usage: (1) humans appear able to create representations from memory that enable them to imagine being in situations purely through mental simulation; (2) the imagining processes can take advantage of affordances in the environment to make problem solving easier; (3) the predictions, and other kinds of solutions arrived at through this kind of mental simulation, are often correct—or good enough—in mundane cases; and (4) when the solution fails, a wide range of culturally available tools can be used, such as getting out a measuring tape or making a calculation.

Recall that the original Craikian notion emphasized the *parallelism* both in form and in operation between external phenomena and internal modeling: "By 'relation-structure' I do not mean some obscure non-physical entity which attends the model, but the fact that it is a physical working model which works in the same way as the process it parallels, in the aspects under consideration at any moment" (Craik 1943, 51). By this I interpret him to mean that the internal model complies with the constraints of the real-world phenomena it represents, not that it is run like a "movie in the head," which signifies vivid and detailed visual representations "running" in real time. Craik based his hypothesis on the need for organisms to be able to predict the environment; thus he saw mental simulation as central to reasoning. He maintained that just as humans create physical models, for example, to experiment with alternatives such as physical-scale models of boats and bridges, so too the nervous system of humans and other organisms has developed a way to create internal " 'small scale model[s]' of external reality" (ibid., 61) for simulating potential outcomes of actions in a physical environment. I interpret his use of quotation marks around "small scale models" to indicate that he meant it figuratively, and not that the brain quite literally creates, for example, an image of a small-scale boat whose motion it simulates as in a movie. He does, however, appear to mean that the representations are modal or perception-based. Mental simulation occurs, he claims, by the "excitation and volley of impulses which parallel the stimuli which occasioned them" (ibid., 60). Thus the internal processes of reasoning result in conclusions similar to those that "might have been reached by causing the actual physical processes to occur" (ibid., 51). In constructing the hypothesis, Craik drew on existing research in neurophysiology and speculated that the ability "to parallel or model external events" (ibid.) is fundamental to the brain.

Modern advocates of mental modeling also speculate that the origins of the capacity lie in a general capacity to simulate possible ways of maneuvering within the physical environment. Since it would be highly adaptive to possess the ability to anticipate the environment and potential outcomes of actions, many organisms should possess the capacity for simulation.[4] Quite conceivably, then, the rat simulates its path through a familiar maze and performs the appropriate actions to get to the food at the end. Given that modern humans have linguistic capabilities, it should be possible to create mental models from both perception and description, which is borne out by the research on narrative and discourse comprehension discussed in the next section. Additionally, studies of expert/novice reasoning lend support to the possibility that skill in mental modeling develops in the course of learning (Chi, Feltovich, and Glaser 1981). The nature and richness of the models one can construct and one's ability to reason develop in learning domain-specific content and techniques. Recent studies show that mental simulation underlies expertise;for example, when sharpshooters imagine shooting a gun, their entire body behaves as if they are actually shooting a gun (Barsalou 1999). Neuroscience research shows that expert performers of a dance form (such as ballet and capoeira), when watching video clips of the dances in which they are experts, show strong activation in premotor, parietal, and posterior STS regions, as compared to when watching other dance forms. Nondancer control participants do not show this effect. Similar motor activation has been shown for expert piano players watching piano playing (Brass and Heyes 2005). In sum, facility with mental modeling is a combination of an individual's biology and learning, and develops in interaction with the natural, social, and cultural realities in which one is embedded.

In the rest of this section I will bring together research on discourse and situation models, mental imagery, mental animation/simulation, and embodied mental representation as providing evidence in support of a Craikian notion of simulative mental modeling.

4.4.1 Discourse and Situation Models

Reading, comprehending, and reasoning about stories would seem to epitomize thinking with language. Yet, there is a significant body of cognitive research that supports the hypothesis that the inferences subjects make from these activities are derived through constructing and manipulating a mental model of the situation depicted by the narrative, rather than by applying rules of inference to a system of propositions representing the content of the text. A major strategy of this approach is to differentiate the structure of the text from the structure of the situation depicted in the text, and investigate which of the structures the cognitive representations follow. Johnson-Laird in psycholinguistics and others in psychology, formal semantics, and linguistics have proposed cognitive representations in the form of working memory "discourse models" or "situation models," which are used in inferences related to narratives. On this proposal, the linguistic expressions assist the reader–listener in constructing a mental model through which he or she understands and reasons about the situation depicted by the narrative. That is, in reasoning, the referent of the text would be an internal model of the situation depicted by the text rather than a description. The central idea is that "discourse models make explicit the structure not of sentences but of situations as we perceive or imagine them" (Johnson-Laird 1989, 471).

The principal tenets of the theory, as outlined by Johnson-Laird, are as follows. As a form of mental model, a discourse model would embody a representation of the spatial, temporal, and causal relationships among the events and entities of the situation described by the narrative. In constructing and updating a model, the reader calls upon a combination of preexisting conceptual and real-world knowledge and employs the tacit and recursive inferencing mechanisms of her cognitive apparatus to integrate the information with that contained in the narrative. In principle these should be able to generate the set of all possible situations a narrative could describe.

A number of experiments have been conducted to investigate the hypothesis that in understanding a narrative readers spontaneously construct mental models to represent and reason about the situations depicted by the text (Dijk and Kintsch 1983; Franklin and Tversky 1990; Johnson-Laird 1983; Mani and Johnson-Laird 1982; McNamara and Sternberg 1983; Morrow, Bower, and Greenspan 1989; Perrig and Kintsch 1985; Zwaan 1999; Zwaan and Radvansky 1998). Although no instructions were given to imagine or picture the situations, when queried about how they had made inferences in response to an experimenter's questioning, most participants reported that it was by means of "seeing" or "being in the situation" depicted. That is, the reader sees herself as an "observer" of a simulated situation. Whether the view of the situation is "spatial" (i.e., a global perspective) or "perspectival" (i.e., from a specific point of view) is still a point of debate, though recent investigations tend to support the perspectival account, that is, the reference frame of the space appears to be that of the body (Bryant and Tversky 1999; Glenberg 1997b; Mainwaring, Tversky, and Schiano 1996).

The interpretation, given these experimental outcomes, is that a situation represented by a mental model could allow the reasoner to generate inferences without having to carry out the extensive operations needed to process the same amount of background information to make inferences from an argument in propositional form.[5] The situational constraints of the narrative are built into the model, making many consequences implicit that would require considerable inferential work to derive in propositional form. Consider, for example, a case where a subject is asked to move an object depicted in a model. Moving an object changes, immediately, its spatial relationships to all the other objects. In simulative mental modeling, the reasoner could grasp this simply by means of the changes in the model and not need to make additional inferences. Such reasoning should be discernibly faster than that of propositional inference. Thus, the reaction time studies noted above provide additional experimental support that making inferences through simulation is faster than making logical inferences from propositions. Finally, reasoning through a model of a situation should restrict the scope of the conclusions drawn. For example, moving an object in a specified manner both limits and makes immediately evident the relevant consequences of that move for other objects in the situation detailed by the narrative. Further support is thus provided by demonstrations in this literature for the claim that it is much more difficult to make inferences—and sometimes they are not made at all—when participants are required to reason with the situation represented in propositional form.

4.4.2 Mental Spatial Simulation

There is an extensive literature that provides evidence that humans can perform various simulative transformations in imagination that mimic physical spatial transformations. The literature on mental imagery establishes that people can mentally simulate combinations. The classic example is of subjects who are asked to imagine a letter B rotated 90 degrees to the left, place an upside triangle below it, and remove the connecting line, to produce an image of a heart. People can perform imaginative rotations that exhibit latencies consistent with actually turning a mental figure around, such as when queried whether two object-representations presented from different rotations are of the same object (Finke 1989; Finke, Pinker, and Farah 1989; Finke and Shepard 1986; Kosslyn 1980, 1994; Shepard and Cooper 1982; Tye 1991), and there is a correlation between the time it takes participants to respond and the number of degrees of rotation required. Further, there is evidence of mental rotational transformations of plane figures and three-dimensional models. As Stephen Kosslyn (1994, 345) summarizes, psychological research provides evidence of rotating, translating, bending, scaling, folding, zooming, and flipping of images. The combinations and transformations in mental imagery are hypothesized to take place according to internalized constraints assimilated during perception (Shepard 1988). Kosslyn also notes that these mental transformations are often accompanied by twisting and moving one's hands to represent rotation, which indicates motor as well as visual processing (see also Jeannerod 1993, 1994; Parsons 1994). Other research indicates that people combine various kinds of knowledge of physical situations with imaginary transformations, including real-time dynamical information (Freyd 1987). When given a problem about objects that are separated by a wall, for instance, the spatial transformations exhibit latencies consistent with the participants having simulated moving around the wall rather than through it, which indicates at least tacit use of physical knowledge that objects cannot move through a wall (Morrow et al. 1989). This kind of knowledge is evidenced in other studies, such as studies in which participants are shown a picture of a person with an arm in front of the body and then one with the arm in back, and they report imagining rotating the arm around the body, rather than through it, and the chronometric measurements are consistent with this (Shiffrar and Freyd 1990).

Although physical knowledge other than spatial appears to be playing a role in such imaginings, it has not been explored systematically in the mental imagery literature. However, as will be discussed below, recent experiments in the ideomotor approach to perception links together imagery, perception, and action (Brass, Bekkering, and Prinz 2002; Brass and Heyes 2005). The kinds of transformations considered thus far are spatial: structural, geometrical, or topological transformations. I refer to the literature on imagery not to make the claim that mental models are like images, but because this literature provides significant evidence for the hypothesis that the human cognitive system is capable of transformative processing in which spatial transformations on iconic representations are made through perceptual and motor processes. Indeed, there is significant evidence from neuropsychology that the perceptual system plays a role in imaginative thinking (see, e.g., Farah 1988; Kosslyn 1994). Again, this makes sense from an evolutionary perspective. The visual cortex is one of the oldest and most highly developed regions of the brain. As Roger Shepard, a psychologist who has done extensive research on visual cognition, has put it, perceptual mechanisms "have, through evolutionary eons, deeply internalized an intuitive wisdom about the way things transform in the world. Because this wisdom is embodied in a perceptual system that antedates, by far, the emergence of language and mathematics, imagination is more akin to visualizing than to talking or to calculating to oneself" (Shepard 1988, 180). Although the original ability to envision, predict, and make inferences by imagining developed as a way of simulating possible courses of action in the world, as humans developed, this ability was "bent to the service of creative thought" (ibid.). Understood in this way, the mundane ability to imagine and visualize underlies some of the most sophisticated forms of human reasoning as evidenced in creative reasoning in science.

Once again, though, the representational format of mental imagery should not be conflated with that of external pictorial representations. As various researchers have shown, for example with Gestalt figures (Chambers and Reisberg 1985), internal representations are more sketchy and less flexible in attempts at reinterpretation. Furthermore, congenitally blind individuals can carry out some classic imagery tasks, though the source of their transformational knowledge is haptic perception and the imagery possibly kinesthetic in nature (Arditi, Holtzman, and Kosslyn 1988; Kerr 1983; Marmor and Zaback 1976).

4.4.3 Mental Animation/Simulation
There is a growing literature in psychology and neuroscience that investigates the hypothesis that the human cognitive system possesses the ability for *mental animation or simulation* in problem-solving tasks.[6] This ability would be central to Craikian mental modeling. Simulative model-based reasoning both in mundane thinking and in science is likely to go beyond just making spatial transformations and extend to the kinds of transformations of physical systems requiring causal and other behavioral knowledge. Indeed, Shepard extended his claim about the nature of the information humans internalize about how things transform in the world to include behavioral constraints, and attempted to develop an account of the psychokinetic laws of such transformations (Shepard 1984, 1994). There is also a significant body of research on infant cognition that has established that days-old infants have an acute sensitivity to causal information. Infants gaze longer and show more interest in events that appear to contradict causality (Spelke 1991; Spelke, Phillips, and Woodward 1995).

Investigations of physical reasoning have moved beyond spatial and temporal transformations to examining the role of causal and behavioral knowledge in mental simulation. An important strand of the mental animation research originates in thinking about the role of diagrammatic representations in reasoning, specifically, inferring motion from static representations. It thus provides insights into the interactions between internal and external representations that we will follow up on in the next section. One indication of interaction is that participants in these kinds of studies often use gestures, sometimes performed over the diagram, that simulate and track the motion (see, e.g., Clement 1994, 2003; Goldin-Meadow et al. 2001; Hegarty and Steinhoff 1997). Prominent research on mental animation includes Hegarty's investigations of reasoning about the behavior of pulley systems (Hegarty 1992; Hegarty and Ferguson 1993; Hegarty and Just 1989) and Daniel Schwartz's studies focusing on gear rotations (Schwartz 1995; Schwartz and Black 1996a,b). These studies, respectively, provide evidence that people are able to perform imaginative causal transformations of configurations of systems of pulleys and of gears when provided with figures of the initial setups. Several findings are important here. Protocols of participants indicate that they do not mentally animate the pulley system all at once as it appears in the real-world experience, but animate it in segments in the causal sequence, working out in a piecemeal fashion the consequences of previous motion for the next segment. The response times for the participants in the gear problems indicate that they, too, animate in sequence, and when given only one set of gears, their response times were proportional to the rate of the angle of rotation.

Participants perform better when given more realistic representations of gears than highly schematic ones, such as those of just circles with no cogs. In the realistic case they seem to make use of tacit physical knowledge, such as of friction, directly to animate the model, whereas in the schematic case they revert to more analytic strategies such as comparing the size of the angles through which gears of different sizes would move. Schwartz's research also indicates that mental animation can make use of other nonvisual information, such as viscosity and gravity. When participants are well trained in rules for inferring motion, however, they often revert to these to solve the problem more quickly (Schwartz and Black 1996a). Mental animation, on the other hand, can result in correct inferences in cases where the participant cannot produce a correct description of the animation (Hegarty 1992). Further, people can judge whether an animation is correct even in cases where the self-produced inference about motion is incorrect (Hegarty 1992).

Another strand of experimental research on mental simulation uses the interference paradigm. For instance, when participants execute an action A (say, tapping fingers on a flat surface), while watching a noncongruent action on a screen (say, an object moving in a direction perpendicular to the tapping) the speed of action A slows down, compared to the condition when the subject is watching a congruent action (Brass, Bekkering, and Prinz 2002). This effect also occurs when only the terminal posture of the noncongruent action is presented on screen. The effect is stronger for actions involving human hands than for actions involving mechanical hands. While doing mental rotation, if participants move their hands or feet in a direction noncompatible with the mental rotation, their performance suffers. Wexler, Kosslyn, and Berthoz (1998) show that unseen motor rotation in the Cooper-Shepard mental rotation task leads to faster reaction times and fewer errors when the motor rotation is compatible with the mental rotation than when it is incompatible. Even planning another action can interfere with mental rotation (Wohlschlager 2001). Supporting these behavioral data is a range of neuroimaging experiments that show that action areas are activated when participants passively watch actions on screen (Brass and Heyes [2005] provide a good review).

A similar process of simulation of actions linked to representations has recently been demonstrated in language understanding. Bergen, Chang, and Narayan (2004) report an imaging study indicating that when participants performed a lexical decision task with verbs referring to actions involving the mouth (like *chew*), leg (like *kick*), or hand (like *grab*), the areas of motor cortex responsible for mouth, leg, or hand motion displayed more activation, respectively. It has also been shown that passive listening to sentences describing mouth, leg, or hand motions activates different parts of the pre-motor cortex. While processing sentences that encode upward motion, like *The ant climbed*, participants take longer to perform a visual categorization task in the upper part of their visual field. The same is true of downward-motion sentences, like *The ant fell*, and the lower half of the visual field. Also, when participants are asked to perform a physical action in response to a sentence, such as moving their hand away from or toward their body, it takes them longer to perform the action if it is incompatible with the motor actions described in the sentence. Extending from these results, the once-criticized motor theory of speech (which argued that perceiving speech involves accessing the speech motor system) is now being reexamined (Galantucci, Fowler, and Turvey 2006).

Two other sources add to the evidence supporting simulation: autonomic responses and neuroimaging experiments (for a comprehensive review, see Svenson and Ziemke 2004). Autonomous response experiments show that responses beyond voluntary control (like heart and respiratory rates) are activated by motor imagery, to an extent proportional to that of actually performing the action. Neuroimaging experiments show that the same brain areas are activated during action and motor imagery of the same action. Gallese et al. (2002) report that when study participants observe goal-related behaviors executed by others (with effectors as different as the mouth, the hand, or the foot) the same cortical sectors are activated as when they perform the same actions. Such studies lead to the conclusion that whenever people look at someone performing an action, in addition to the activation of various visual areas, there is a concurrent activation of the motor circuits that are recruited when they perform that action, themselves. People do not overtly reproduce the observed action, but the motor system acts as if they were executing the same action they are observing. This effect exists in monkeys as well, and such motor-area activation results even with abstract stimuli, such as when a monkey just hears the sound of a peanut cracking. This effect has been replicated across a series of studies (see particularly the work on mirror neurons and canonical neurons; Hurley and Chater [2005a,b] provide a good review).

Although not much research has been conducted with scientists, what there is indicates that they, too, perform mental simulation in problem solving (Clement 1994; Trafton, Trickett, and Mintz, 2005). As with the gear and pulley studies, this research provides evidence of significant interaction between internal and external representations in mental simulation. Though it is some distance from employing causal transformations of rotating gears or pulleys to employing the kinds of transformations requiring scientific knowledge, the mental animation research supports the position that the scientific practices originate in and develop out of mundane imaginative simulation abilities.

4.4.4 Internal–External Coupling

As noted previously, mental modeling is often carried out in the presence of real-world resources, including representations such as diagrams and objects such as sofas. One reason why taking external resources into account is important is that the possibility of simulative reasoning in anything but the simplest of cases is often disparaged as requiring representations and processing much too detailed and complex to be "in the head." How might the mental capability interface with relevant resources in the external world? Much of the research on this question is directed toward diagrams and other kinds of visual representations. Research by Jiajie Zhang (Zhang 1997; Zhang and Norman 1995), for instance, analyzes diagrams as external representations that are coupled as an information source with the individual solving problems. Recently, Hegarty has argued that the corpus of research on mental animation in the context of visual representations leads to the conclusion that internal and external representations are best seen as forming a "coupled system" (Hegarty 2005). In considering the relation between mental modeling and external physical models, I, too, have argued in favor of "internal–external representational coupling" (Nersessian 2005; Nersessian et al. 2003).

As discussed earlier, on the traditional cognitive science view, reasoning uses information abstracted from the external environment and represented and processed internally. Various sorts of information displayed in the world might assist working memory by, for example, colocating information that gets abstracted (Larkin 1989; Larkin and Simon 1987), but all cognitive processing is internal to the individual mind. As discussed in chapter 1, the traditional view is under challenge by several current cognitive research strands that reconstrue "representation" to comprise information remaining in the environment and "processing" to take place within the coupled system linking internal and external worlds. An influential study promoting this view showed that in the Tetris video game, players use actions in the world to lower internal computational load—what the researchers call "epistemic actions" (Kirsh and Maglio 1994). Tetris involves maneuvering falling shapes ("zoids") into specific arrangements on the screen. Players execute actions on the falling zoids, to expose information early, to prime themselves to recognize zoids faster, and to perform external checks and verifications to reduce the uncertainty of judgments. Gestures during cognitive tasks have been shown to lower cognitive load and promote learning (Goldin-Meadow and Wagner 2005). Kirsh (1995) reports higher accuracy in a coin-counting task when participants pointed at the stimulus, compared to a no-pointing condition. Additionally, humans and other animals exploit head and eye movements to better perceive depth, absolute distance, heading, and three-dimensional objects (Wexler and van Boxtel 2005).

Generally speaking, there is a growing recognition that mundane and scientific problem-solving practices indicate the need to consider anew the relationship between the internal and external worlds, so that they are understood as forming a coupled *cognitive system*. On this view, inferences are made by the cognitive system, which comprises people and a range of artifacts. In the case of science, evidence from historical records, protocols, and ethnographic observations of "science in action" establishes that many kinds of external representations are used in model-based reasoning: linguistic (descriptions, narratives, written and oral communications), mathematical equations, visual representations, gestures, physical models, and computational models. Thus the cognitive systems of scientific practice need to be understood as incorporating a wide range of representations and physical resources in problem-solving processes. Although this is not the context in which to consider these perspectives in depth (see Nersessian 2005 for a more extended discussion), it is important to have a flavor of the position to understand the model-based reasoning processes in terms of the coupled system notion.

From an environmental perspective, the environment does not simply "scaffold" cognitive processes as on traditional accounts; rather, aspects of the environment are held to be integral in the cognitive system and thus to enter essentially into the analysis of cognition. Explanations of human cognitive processing in this area often employ the notion of "attunement to constraints and affordances," adapted from J. J. Gibson's (1979) theory of perception. On the *situative* adaptation (Greeno 1998), an "affordance" is a resource in the environment that supports an activity, and a "constraint" is a regularity in a domain that is dependent on specific conditions. The structure of an environment provides constraints and affordances needed in problem solving, including other people. The more radical among the proponents of this view hold that cognitive processing requires only external constraints and affordances; there is no need for internal representations. Given the complexity of some human reasoning, and scientific reasoning in particular, solving many kinds of problems without internal representations seems as implausible as solving them without external resources. The major problem that needs to be resolved in future research is the nature of the cognitive mechanisms through which the internal and external worlds mesh. On the one hand, given that some mental simulation can take place in the absence of external stimuli, the mechanisms need to be such as to take stored information and process it in such a way as to allow for the possibility of at least some of the same inferences as if the real-world stimuli were present. On the other hand, as Daniel Dennett has noted succinctly, "[j]ust as you cannot do very much carpentry with your bare hands, there's not much thinking you can do with your bare mind" (Dennett 2000, 17). In the case at hand, we are considering what the scientific mind needs to carry out creative reasoning.

In the modeling practices of science, the internal and external worlds can be conceived as forming a cognitive system that jointly carries out model-based reasoning. The primary mantra of the distributed and situated research is that cognition is not only "in the mind" or "in the world" but "in the system" such that an individual's mental activities comprise interactions with other material and informational systems (including other humans). To accommodate this insight, the distributed cognition perspective proposes analyses of cognitive processing that incorporate the *salient* resources in the environment in a nonreductive fashion (see, e.g., Hutchins 1995a,b; Norman 1991). Salient resources are, broadly characterized, those factors in the environment that can affect the outcome of a cognitive activity, such as problem solving. These cannot be determined a priori but need to be judged with respect to the instance. For ship navigators, for example, the function of a specific instrument would be salient to piloting the ship, but the material from which the instrument is made would typically not be. For physicists, whether one sketches on a blackboard or whiteboard or piece of paper is likely irrelevant to solving a problem; but sketching on a computer screen has the potential to be salient because the computer adds resources that can affect the outcome.

The artifacts of a culture that perform cognitive functions are referred to as "cognitive artifacts," and determining these within a specific system is a major part of the analytical task for environment-driven cognition. Hutchins has studied the cognitive contributions of artifacts employed in modern navigation, such as the alidade, gyrocompass, and fathometer. Various kinds of external representations are candidate cognitive artifacts, and much research has focused on visual representations, especially diagrams. In addition to the mental animation literature discussed above, there is an extensive literature on diagrammatic representations that reinforces the "coupled system" notion, such as that of Zhang and Norman referenced earlier. They have studied problem solving with isomorphic problems to ascertain potential cognitive functions of different kinds of visual representations and have found that external representations differentially facilitate and constrain reasoning processes. The format of the external representation, for example, can change the nature of the processing task, as when the tic-tac-toe grid is imposed on the mathematical problem of "15." Specifically, they argue that diagrams can play more than just a supportive role in what is essentially an internal process; rather, these external representations can be coupled directly as an information source with the person, without requiring the mediation of an internal representation of the information provided in them. Not all external representations are equally facilitating, though, as Bauer and Johnson-Laird (1993) show in their study of diagrams in mental modeling tasks. Intriguingly, diagrams with information represented with amodal tokens appear to provide no facilitation, but diagrams with symbols perceptually resembling the objects being reasoned about (modal tokens) do significantly enhance problem solving, as was evidenced also in the mental animation research.

Research on problem solving with diagrammatic representations in formal logic by Keith Stenning and colleagues shows that diagrams restrict the internal problem space so as to constrain the kinds of inferences that can be made (Stenning 2002; Stenning and Oberlander 1995). Recently, Trafton and colleagues (Trafton, Trickett, and Mintz 2005) investigated scientists' interactions with computer visualizations, which offer more and greater ease of possibilities for manipulation during problem solving. They found that in the presence of external computer visualizations, scientists tend to do considerable mental manipulations, interacting with the visualization represented before them, instead of either just creating a mental image or making direct adjustments to the image on the computer screen. Their manipulations and comparisons appear to be aimed at constructing a mental model constrained by the computer visualization, but through which the implications of the visualization could be understood.

The ethnographic studies my research group has been conducting examine the role of representations in the form of physical devices that are models constructed by biomedical engineers for simulating *in vivo* biological processes. Within the cognitive systems in the laboratory these physical devices instantiate part of the current community model of the phenomena and allow simulation and manipulation of this understanding. One researcher we studied aptly referred to the process of constructing and manipulating these *in vitro* physical models as "putting a thought into the bench top and seeing whether it works or not." These instantiated "thoughts" allow researchers to perform controlled simulations of an *in vivo* context, for example, of the local forces at work in the artery. We interpret such simulative model-based reasoning as a process of co-constructing and manipulating the "internal" researcher models of the phenomena and of the device and the "external" model that is the device, each incomplete. In this context, simulative model-based reasoning would consist of processing information both in memory and in the environment (see also Gorman 1997; Greeno 1989). Although the capacity for making inferences might be ascribed to the traditionally conceived "mental" part, the internal and external representations and processes involved in simulative model-based reasoning are best understood as a coupled system. Thus the ascription of "mental" might better be construed as pertaining more to the property that inferences are generated from it than to it as a locus or medium of operation. Components of the inferential system would include both one or more people and artifacts (Osbeck and Nersessian 2006).

One way to accommodate the hypothesis of coupling between external and internal representations is to expand the notion of memory to encompass external representations and cues; that is, to construe specific kinds of affordances and constraints in the environment, literally, as memory in cognitive processing. If memory is so distributed, then we can conceive of the *problem space* not in the traditional way as internally represented, but as comprising internal and external resources (Nersessian 2005; Nersessian et al. 2003). The evolutionary psychologist Merlin Donald (Donald 1991) has argued that evolutionary considerations lead to the view that human memory encompasses internal and external representation. Donald uses a wide range of evidence from anthropology, archeology, primatology, and neuroscience to argue his case. He maintains that this evidence establishes that external representations have been and continue to be indispensable to complex human thinking, and their development was central to the processes of cultural transmission. Donald's analysis of the evolutionary emergence of distinctively human representational systems starts from the significance of mimesis—such as using the body to represent an idea of the motion of an airplane—in the developments of such external representations as painting and drawing (40,000 years ago), writing (6,000 years ago), and phonetic alphabets (4,000 years ago). The artifacts that contribute to remembering are social and cultural constructs designed by human communities that rely on them in supporting remembering. Donald argues for a distributed notion of memory as a symbiosis of internal and external representation on the basis of changes in the visuo-spatial architecture of human cognition that came about with the development of external representation. On this notion, affordances and constraints in the environment are *ab initio* part of cognitive processing.

As noted, recasting cognition such that the relationship between the internal and external worlds form a coupled cognitive-cultural system presents cognitive scientists with the challenge of determining the mechanisms of representation and processing that would enable this coupling. Greeno sets the criteria that the internal representations in mental modeling processes be such that "we interact with them in ways that are similar to our interactions with physical and—probably—social environments" (Greeno 1989, 313), and thus be such that they are "acquired with significant properties of external situations and one's interactions with the situations . . . such that at least some of the properties are known implicitly in something like the way that we know how to interact with [external] environments" (ibid., 314). These requirements echo the earlier views of Craik, as do the analyses of Shepard (1984, 1988, 1994) on the internalization of physical constraints. Human representations need also to be such that they interface smoothly with the other system representations in problem-solving processes. One plausible way for making the interfacing "smooth" is for human representations to have modal aspects such that perceptual and motor mechanisms are employed in cognitive processing.

4.4.5 Embodied Mental Representation: "Perceptual" Mental Models

What might the format of the representation of a "Craikian" mental model be? For Johnson-Laird's analysis of logical reasoning, that the working memory constructs are amodal iconic, as discussed earlier, perhaps suffices for logical reasoning. Model-based reasoning about physical systems, however, needs to allow simulations of physical entities, situations, and processes that go beyond manipulating amodal tokens in a spatial array.

Following Craik's notion of parallelism in the form and operation of representations used in reasoning, working memory models of physical systems would be perception-based representations. Considerable knowledge would be needed for such a mental simulation, not just what can be derived from perception as it is usually understood as separate from conceptual understanding. The behaviors of the parts of the model, for example, need to be connected to knowledge of how these function, although much of it can be tacit. To take a simple example, people can usually infer how water will spill out of a cup without being able to make explicit or describe the requisite knowledge. Although we have only been considering mental modeling as a working memory process, of course information from long-term memory plays a role in this process. Mental modeling representations need to maintain a connection to long-term memory representations, and so an account is needed of how information might be stored so as to connect to working memory representations.

It is a commonsense observation that humans do have some means of storing knowledge and of calling it selectively into use, but the format of that information remains an open question. In this section I draw on research on *embodied* representations in support of the notion that information contained in working memory representation could be modal. The modal aspect would likely facilitate representational coupling in reasoning processes, and most likely, some of the information to which the models are connected in memory, enabling simulation, also has a modal aspect. The embodied representation research focuses on the implications of the interaction of the human perceptual system with the environment for internal representation and processing, generally. Proponents contend that a wide range of empirical evidence shows that perceptual content is retained in all kinds of mental representations, and that perceptual and motor mechanisms of the brain play a significant role in many kinds of cognitive processing traditionally conceived as separate from these, including memory, conceptual processing, and language comprehension (see, e.g., Barsalou 1999, 2003; Barsalou et al. 2003; Barsalou, Solomon, and Wu 1999; Catrambone, Craig, and Nersessian 2005; Craig, Nersessian, and Catrambone 2002a,b; Glenberg 1997b; Johnson 1987; Kosslyn 1994; Lakoff 1987; Solomon and Barsalou 2004; Yeh and Barsalou 1996).

One extensive area of research concerns the representation of spatial information in mental models. This research leads to the conclusion that internal representation of spatial configurations does not provide an "outsider" three-dimensional Euclidian perspective—the "view from nowhere"—but provides an embodied version that is relative to the orientation of one's body and to gravity. In early research Irwin Rock hypothesized that there is a "deeply ingrained tendency to 'project' egocentric up-down, left-right coordinates onto the [imagined] scene" (Rock 1973, 17). This hypothesis is borne out by recent research (see, e.g., Bryant and Tversky 1999; Bryant, Tversky, and Franklin 1992; Franklin and Tversky 1990; Glenberg 1997a; Perrig and Kintsch 1985). In particular, Barbara Tverksy and colleagues have found that mental spatial alignment corresponds with bodily sym-metry—up-down, front-back, and gravity—depending on how the partici-pant is oriented in the external environment. When the participant is asked to imagine objects surrounding an external central object, mental model alignment depends on whether the object has the same orientation as the observer. This bodily orientation could be tied to preparation for *situated action* paralleling that which would occur in real-world situations (Glenberg 1997a).

A second line of research focuses on concept representation. From an embodied cognition alternative, a "concept is a neural structure that is actually part of, or makes use of, the sensorimotor system of our brains" (Lakoff and Johnson 1998, 20). As we saw, in traditional cognitive-science theories of representation, concepts are represented by amodal, language-like structures, including definitions, feature lists of prototypes, and frames. Reasoning is carried out on these by means of manipulations such as allowed by logic, condition-action rules, and domain-specific rules. Here again the influence of the literal interpretation of the mind–computer analogy is evident, since these kinds of information structures and pro-cesses comprise those that can be implemented on computers. We are now in a period where neuroscience has advanced to the point that the differ-ences between the brain and the computer are coming to the fore, and where differences between the human–environment relationship and the computer–environment relationship are under consideration in theorizing about the nature of cognitive representations and processes. Just how the mental models would be "run" in simulative reasoning is an open research question requiring more knowledge about the cognitive and neural mecha-nisms underlying such processes. But it cannot be assumed a priori that these reduce to the same kinds of computations assumed by AI researchers. And, even if deductive and inductive reasoning were to use amodal repre-sentations, it is possible that simulative reasoning could involve modal representations and call on perceptual–motor mechanisms.

Among others, Lawrence Barsalou has been formulating an account (first fully articulated in Barsalou 1999) of the human conceptual system that calls into question the traditional understanding of concept representation as amodal. A wide range of research dovetails in thinking about embodiment and representation, but I will focus largely on the recent work of Barsalou and colleagues because they argue for the perceptual basis of concept representation through drawing together evidence from much of that research, as well as through experiments specifically designed to test the hypothesis. Since my goal is not to argue that Barsalou's theory is "right"—but rather to advocate that it goes in the right direction for further articulating the kind of account of simulative model-based reasoning the science case requires—I present only the broad outlines.

Barsalou argues and convincingly demonstrates that there is an extensive experimental literature that can be read as supporting the contention that mental representations retain perceptual features, and that many cognitive functions involve the reenactment or "simulation" of perceptual states. These include perceptual processing, memory, language, categorization, and inference. He makes a compelling experimental case for the broad claims of the theory from evidence drawn from existing behavioral and neuroscience research, and behavioral tasks designed specifically to test its implications (summarized in Barsalou 2003). The experiments he and his colleagues have designed to test the implications of the theory primarily involve property generation and property verification tasks. They distinguish between the alternatives of simulating the referent of a word (modal version) and looking up a word in a semantic network or frame (amodal version). The participants are given either a neutral condition with no instructions on how to do the task or an imagery condition where they are asked to visualize or imagine the referent. On the amodal version, the neutral condition should produce patterns of response different from the imagery condition. Across a wide range of terms, these experiments show a similar pattern of responses between the two conditions, favoring the modal version. Other significant experiments involve manipulating perceptual variables, such as occlusion. For example, in property-generation experiments, participants listed twice as many internal features of objects when they were presented with modified object terms, such as "rolled-up lawn" (e.g., roots) as opposed to "lawn," "½ watermelon" (e.g., seeds), and "glass car" (e.g., seats) (Barsalou et al. 2003; Barsalou et al. 1999). Experiments using fMRI in the neutral condition provide evidence of activity in sensorimotor areas of the brain during the property-generation task, whereas on the traditional separation of cognition and perception (amodal version), there should be no activation in sensorimotor areas when representing a concept (Simmons et al. 2004).

On Barsalou's modal account, cognitive processing employs "perceptual symbols," which are neural correlates of sensorimotor experiences (Barsalou 1999). These symbols "result from an extraction process that selects some subset of a perceptual state and stores it as a symbol" (Barsalou and Prinz 1997, 275). Perceptual symbols can be created from introspection as well, such as through abstractive processes. The relationship between the symbols and what they represent is analogical, as opposed to arbitrary. The perceptual symbols form a common representational system that underlies both sensorimotor and conceptual processing. Because the conceptual system makes use of perceptual and motor mechanisms, concept representations are distributed across modality-specific systems. These representations possess simulation capabilities; that is, perceptual and motor processes associated with the original experiences are reenacted when perceptual symbols are employed in thinking. Concepts are separable neural states underlying perception and constituting the units of long-term memory representation, which in turn can be organized into knowledge units such as schemas, mental models, or frames.

Connections among various representations are made during categorization processes, including the construction of ad hoc categories, to form "perceptual symbol systems." One strong objection against perceptual representations has been that they cannot accommodate properties known to hold of conceptual systems, such as the potential to produce an infinite number of conceptual combinations and the capability to distinguish types from tokens and to represent abstract concepts. The need to accommodate these known possibilities of conceptual representations led to the traditional propositional (amodal) account, rather than direct empirical evidence in favor of it. However, there are several notorious problems with the amodal account, including the "symbol grounding problem," that is, the problem of how the arbitrary transductions are mapped back onto perceptual states and entities in the world (Harnad 1990; Searle 1980). Barsalou (1999) and, later, Jesse Prinz (Prinz 2002) provided arguments that, in principle, perceptual symbol systems can exhibit all the salient characteristics of propositional systems. The (mis-)perception that they cannot stems from the tendency to conflate perceptual symbol systems with *recording systems* in which images are captured but not interpreted (Haugeland 1991). Performing a perceptual simulation is not akin to "running" a kind of motion picture in the head. The human conceptual system is interpretive and inferential. Perceptual symbols are not holistic representations of their real-world counterparts, and their componential, schematic, and dynamic nature allows for combination, recombination, and abstraction. Barsalou, too, stresses that the human conceptual system should not be understood by means of an analogy to a recording system. Perceptual symbols are schematic extractions from perceptual processes that allow for infinite possibilities of imaginative recombination. Further, one should not expect simulations to be as detailed or vivid as the original perceptions. In conducting a perceptual simulation, one need be consciously aware of neither mental imagery, which requires extra cognitive effort to produce, nor the simulation process.

There are many open questions about modal representation for which only partial solutions have been suggested, such as: How do abstract concepts become represented? How does "translation" take place across modalities? How does integration take place? And, how are perceptually dissimilar instances of a concept recognized and categorized? But there are many open questions about amodal representation as well, and, significantly, as Barsalou points out, there is little direct empirical evidence in favor of a fully amodal view. In sum, Barsalou and other proponents of embodied cognition do make a compelling case that at the very least a more tempered conclusion is warranted in the present circumstances, and this is sufficient for our needs: "The conceptual system appears neither fully modular nor fully amodal. To the contrary, it is non-modular in sharing many important mechanisms with perception and action. Additionally it traffics heavily in the modal representations that arise in sensory-motor systems" (Barsalou 2003, 27). Thus, how modal representations could contribute to various cognitive processes, such as mental modeling, merits investigation.

The point I want to make from this research is that a working memory model with modal iconic aspects (which I will now call a "perceptual mental model") better fits the simulation needs for reasoning about physical systems, as well as the need for interfacing between external and internal representations. Concept representation is likely to have both modal and amodal aspects. The modal aspects serve the requirements of simulative mental modeling we have been discussing. Recall that on Craik's speculation, mental simulation occurs by the "excitation and volley of impulses which parallel the stimuli which occasioned them" (Craik 1943, 60), with simulative reasoning processes resulting in conclusions similar to those that "might have been reached by causing the actual physical processes to occur" (ibid., 51). On the perceptual symbol theory, too, the human conceptual system is predicated on a form of reenactment, where working-memory-specific concept representations are constructed for the purpose of supporting situated action. One important implication of the modal view of category representation is that, rather than being context-free, object representations include situational information that is active in conceptual processing. There is abundant empirical evidence from psychological experiments favoring this implication (Yeh and Barsalou 1996), which supports the idea that the conceptual system is "organized around the action-environment interface" (Barsalou 2003, 12). In situated action, "a concept is a skill that delivers specialized packages of inferences to guide an agent's interactions with specific category members in particular situations. Across different situations, different packages tailor inferences to different goals and situational constraints" (ibid., 27). Thus, to have a concept is to possess a skill for constructing a potentially infinite number of simulations tailored to one's immediate goals and needs for action.

If we conceive of simulative model-based reasoning about physical systems as a form of "situated action," it allows the reasoning to be fully imaginative or to be carried out in conjunction with real-world action, such as looking at the sofa and the doorway when reasoning, drawing a sketch or diagram, or using a physical device to simulate a model. Mental modeling in conjunction with external resources form a coupled system by which inferences are made. In this way the problem solver does not simply "use" external representations; rather, they are incorporated directly into the *cognitive* processing. Such a notion of mental modeling would meet Greeno's criteria that people should be able to interact with the internal representations "in ways that are similar to our interactions with physical and—probably—social environments" (Greeno 1989, 313). Perceptual mental models are built on representations "acquired with significant properties of external situations and one's interactions with the situations . . . such that at least some of the properties are known implicitly in something like the way that we know how to interact with [external] environments" (ibid., 314). Affordances and constraints of situational information, thus, would be at play even in the solely imaginative cases of mental modeling where only one's conceptual understanding is used.

Stephen Kosslyn's (1994) theory of imagery manipulation provides a possible way of thinking about the construction and manipulation of working memory mental models and their relation to information in long-term memory. On Kosslyn's account, images are not manipulated in the visual buffer. Rather, they are manipulated "off-line" by means of links to information in long-term memory, and the image is updated in the visual buffer after that processing has taken place. On Barsalou's account, long-term memory representations are linked to neural states arising from perception. If perceptual mental models constructed in working memory retain their connections to the long-term representations and were manipulated in a way similar to Kosslyn's account of imagery, this could mitigate concerns about working memory limitations for simulation and also be consistent with the notion that processing is piecemeal, as is supported by the mental animation literature referenced previously.

Barsalou's research considers internal concepts, how they encode perceptual and motor elements, and how these elements are triggered in using the concepts. It does not consider, however, how external objects and traces trigger the perceptual and motor elements—which is needed for the notion of coupling. It could account for this possibility by arguing that perception of affordances triggers internal actions linked to the affordances, just as a linguistic trigger would, but his theory has not considered this point until now. Recent research within a growing theoretical movement termed "ideomotor theory" provides a start on how to think about internal–external coupling. The movement locates its prehistory in a observation by William James:

Every representation of a movement awakens in some degree the actual movement which is its object; and awakens it in a maximum degree whenever it is not kept from doing so by an antagonistic representation present simultaneously in the mind. (James 1890)

Accounts that draw on this idea postulate that brain states automatically mimic movements in the world (Brass and Heyes 2005; Prinz 2005). This automatic activation of movement by perception is considered usually to stay covert as a result of inhibition, but the covert simulation of movement is thought to contribute toward cognitive processes. Researchers interpret the experimental data to mean both that internal simulation can be supported by external stimuli with dynamic properties and also that it can be hindered by them, if the internal and external are not in accord. Internal activation can be triggered by perceptual affordances and by linguistic stimuli. In effect, the body resonates to external movement, and to external stimuli that encode/afford movement, such as in the example of monkey and peanut noted earlier (Metzinger and Gallese 2003). The possibility that even static stimuli trigger simulation could enable the coupling between internal and static external representations, such as diagrams, in mental modeling.

4.5   Mental Modeling and Scientific Model-based Reasoning Practices

To summarize the argument of this chapter, mental modeling is a fundamental form of human reasoning. It evolved as an efficient means of navigating the environment and solving problems significant for surviving in the world. Humans have extended its use to more esoteric situations, such as constructing scientific representations. My analysis of model-based reasoning in conceptual change requires only the adoption of a "minimalist" mental modeling hypothesis: in certain problem-solving tasks, people reason by constructing an internal iconic model of the situations, events, and processes that in dynamic cases can be manipulated through simulation. Such a mental model is an organized unit of knowledge that embodies representations of spatiotemporal relations, representations of situations, entities, and processes, as well as representations of other pertinent information, such as causal structure. Reasoning is carried out by means of model construction and manipulation. In the processes of constructing, manipulating, and revising mental models, information in various formats, including linguistic, formulaic, visual, auditory, and kinesthetic, can be used to construct and animate the model. The interaction with external representations during reasoning, which I cast as representational coupling, led to the notion that mental models in working memory have significant modal aspects ("perceptual mental model"), though a conclusive argument for or against this cannot be made from either the modal or amodal literatures.

How does this notion of mental modeling as simulative reasoning relate to the exemplars of reasoning practices in the sciences? My account casts the specific conceptual changes as arising from iterative processes of constructing, manipulating, evaluating, and revising analog models to satisfy constraints. Cognitive-historical analysis casts the scientific practices as deriving from the cognitive capacity for mental modeling. A mental model is a conceptual system representing the physical system that is being reasoned about. As such, it is an abstraction—idealized and schematic in nature—that represents a physical situation by having surrogate objects and properties, relations, behaviors, or functions of these that are in correspondence with it. The S2 think-aloud protocol provides ample evidence of Craik's notion that mental models parallel physical systems—what I have interpreted as the iconic nature of the mental representations. It also provides evidence for the coupled interaction between internal and external representation in reasoning processes, of reasoning through model simulation, and of perceptual inferencing more generally. Although the Maxwell case does not derive from data that aimed to make his thinking processes explicit, he too drew iconic external representations, made inferences through manipulating them, and, in published work, provided the reader with instructions for mentally animating these representations. Both provide evidence that mental models interact with external representations—diagrams (drawn by S2 and Maxwell), written equations (Maxwell's derivations), verbal representations such as written (Maxwell's instructions for simulating the lines in three dimensions as extending out of the flat page) or oral descriptions (S2's comments about having a visual image immediately prior to drawing a figure), and gestural representations (S2's simulation of the motion of a spring or rod with his hands) provide examples of these representations. On the account developed in this chapter, mental models embody and comply with the constraints of the phenomena being reasoned about, and thus enable inferences about these phenomena through simulation processes. Examples of constraints include causal coherence (Maxwell introduces the idle wheels to eliminate the friction problem) and consistency, both physical consistency (S2's rod model should stretch with constant slope as does the spring) and mathematical consistency (Maxwell's mathematical representation of field needs to be consistent with Ampère's law). Inferences made in the simulation processes provided each with new data that played a role in evaluating and adapting models to comply with the new constraints (such as the droop of a bending rod for S2 and the jamming of vortices for Maxwell).

That genuine reasoning can take place through constructing and manipulating models helps to make sense of much of scientific practice that has been neglected by historians or ruled as insignificant by philosophers. As discussed in chapter 1, traditional philosophical accounts view reasoning as carrying out logical operations on propositional representations. Philosophers are beginning to recognize the significance of modeling as a creative engine driving scientific discovery and change, in part owing to the pervasive and growing use of computer modeling and simulation by contemporary scientists, but there is scant research on the intellectual work carried out with models. In developing the computational practices, however, scientists are using new instrumentation to enrich and take to new depths and directions an existing human practice: simulative model-based reasoning. The situation parallels such developments as those of the telescope, microscope, and other instrumentation that have enabled scientists to "see" better. Computer modeling (as well as modeling with physical simulations) enables scientists to "simulate" better. But just as with those instruments, there is no need to claim that what the humans do in model-based reasoning—the representations they use and the nature of the processing—is anything like what the computers do.

In a look ahead to chapter 6, I now sketch how mental modeling provides a cognitive basis for creativity in conceptual change. The core idea is that abstractive processes in model construction enable integration of information from multiple sources specific to the problem-solving situation, which allows truly novel combinations to emerge as candidate solutions to representational problems. What is powerful about this idea is that constraints abstracted from different sources can interact in such a way that a model with a heretofore unrepresented structure or behaviors can emerge, as we saw in the historically creative Maxwell exemplar and the personally creative S2 exemplar. The results of these recombinations can be explored imaginatively—alone or in conjunction with physical realizations—and through expression in other representational formats, such as mathematics and language. To understand more how recombinations can come about, we will take a look in chapter 5 at the reasoning modalities of analogy, imagery, and thought-experimenting used in conceptual change. The new twists I give on these are that analogies are cast as sources of constraints for building models, that imagistic representations afford simulative reasoning, and, as should be obvious from this chapter, that thought-experimenting is construed as a form of reasoning through imaginative simulation.

5 Representation and Reasoning: Analogy, Imagery, Thought Experiment

The words or the language, as they are written or spoken, do not seem to play any role in my mechanism of thought. The psychical entities which seem to serve as elements in thought are certain signs and more or less clear images which can be "voluntarily" reproduced and combined . . . this combinatory play seems to be the essential feature in productive thought before there is any connection with logical construction in words or other kinds of signs which can be communicated to others.

—Albert Einstein, in a letter to Jacques Hadamard, quoted in *The Creative Process*

With the notion of mental modeling as simulative model-based reasoning in hand, I now address the question: How are mental models created, manipulated, evaluated, and adapted in problem-solving processes? Answering this question brings us back to a central observation discussed in chapter 1: the use of analogies, thought experiments, and imagistic representations figures prominently in creative problem solving across the sciences, often leading to conceptual innovation. As we saw in the historical exemplar, Maxwell's use of these in creating, investigating, and modifying a series of models achieved a radical reconceptualization of electromagnetic phenomena. One significant aspect common to these modes of thinking is that they all involve ways of changing representations, by which I mean the following. Making an analogy, for instance, can involve changes that enable understanding one representation in terms of another. An analogy between an atom and the solar system, for instance, requires each representation to be re-represented more abstractly as a centrally located entity around which other entities orbit. Once this is done, one can then examine to what extent problem solutions in the solar system domain, such as the inverse square law for forces between the entities, transfer to the atom. In making an analogy between magnetism and continuum mechanics, Maxwell represented the magnetic forces as

motions of vortices in an elastic fluid medium. Although no ready-to-hand
solution for the kinds of problems he was investigating existed in continuum mechanics, making the transformation allowed him to tap a range of
representational resources of that domain, especially the mathematical
representations of continuum phenomena, and ultimately to use them to
represent electromagnetism.

Imagistic representation can involve many different kinds of transformations. Some kinds of imagistic representation involve change in format,
such as changing a propositional representation into a visual one. The
claim that "a face is like a car," for instance, might only be intelligible
through visually representing a car schematically with prominent head-
lights (eyes), grill (nose), and bumper (mouth) as in cartoons. Another type
of change through imagistic representation is creating an external visualization of an internal imagining. S2's sketches of what he was imagining,
for instance, enabled manipulating the mental representation more easily.
Through highlighting features they facilitated noticing more readily the
consequences of imagining, such as the possible motions of an object
drawn in a sketch. Gestures, too, can be interpreted as transforming internal representations to external imagistic representations, such as when S2
gestured the motion of his imagined models.

Finally, a thought experiment is a form of mental simulation that
involves constructing a representation and then changing it through imagining future states. Einstein, for example, constructed a model of a physicist in a chest being pulled with constant acceleration in outer space. In
imagining the potential effects of that motion (changes of state) given that
representation, he established that the effects in the moving chest would
be the same as if the physicist were stationary in a gravitational field.
Thought experiments need not be elaborate formulations conveyed in
stories, as are the familiar famous exemplars. They can consist simply in
"as if" experimental reasoning, such as asking the question "What would
happen if . . . ?" and making the corresponding changes in the representation. Maxwell, for instance, in conceiving of what would happen if the
magnetic vortices were in motion in a medium, noticed the problem of
friction. S2, imagining what would happen if the hexagonal spring were
being stretched, noticed there would be a twisting motion in the line segments. In previous work, I have argued that traditional thought experiments belong to the same class of conceptual simulations as this kind of
imaginative reasoning (Nersessian 1991, 1992a,b).

In mundane cases a mental model might be assembled fairly easily from
familiar representations in memory, even in the case of imaginary models,

such as of pink elephants flying. What is notable in our exemplars is not just that the models are imaginary, but the nature of the considerable intellectual work that was required to bring together the representational resources to create a model through which to reason. In the Maxwell case, the requisite representation for solving the electromagnetic problems outstrips the current community resources, and, for S2, his existing representation of a spring does not include the needed representation of torsion. Each case involves creating a series of analog models embodying constraints from both the target phenomena and the analogical source domain. One reason I developed the exemplars in terms of constraints was to make explicit the contributions of target, source, and model to creating and evaluating the adequacy of each model. Another is that I think it affords a new way of understanding conceptual innovation, as will be discussed in chapter 6. In chapters 2 and 3 we saw that the constructed models are imaginary hybrids of target and source domains, possessing constraints of their own as well. Once a constructed model was established to be an adequate representation, the inferences that flow from it could be transferred to the target problem. This kind of iterative problem solving fits the metaphor of a *bootstrapping* process. Each constructed model is built upon the previous model, based on the evaluation of how well that model fits the target phenomena and the enhanced understanding of the target the evaluation provides. The evaluation can yield new constraints that the next model in the processes needs to satisfy. Figures 2.17 and 3.16 are schematic representations of the bootstrapping processes of Maxwell and S2, respectively.

This chapter focuses on the roles of analogy, imagery, and imaginative simulation in such bootstrapping processes. As noted in the discussion of mental modeling, creative scientific practices are of far greater complexity and sophistication than any of those studied in current psychological investigations and cannot be explained by reducing them to psychological theories or computational implementations based on the experimental studies. Nevertheless, the cognitive science literature does provide important insights for my account, and these will be discussed in the context of how they relate to scientific model-based reasoning practices. Once again, we can place the scientific practices on a continuum with how people use these modes of reasoning to solve more ordinary problems, and, reflexively, raise considerations stemming from the creative reasoning practices of scientists for which cognitive research is not yet sufficient to explain.

One major source of insufficiency is that in the cognitive literature the mundane practices are largely investigated separately in different areas of research. To a significant extent, separation is necessary given the goals and methods of cognitive psychology. Standard laboratory experiments need to be conducted in a limited time frame, manipulating a tractable number of variables and aiming to develop quantifiable measures of cognitive processes. The real-world practices of scientists, however, provide numerous instances for which such division is artificial and both calls into question that separation for developing cognitive theories and affords an opportunity for thinking about integration. Take, for instance, the simple analogy Galileo made between the motion of a stone dropped from the mast of a moving ship and the motion of a ball dropped from a tower on the Earth. This analogy functions also as a thought experiment. Or consider Newton's analogy between the motion of a projectile thrown with successively greater velocity from a mountain rising high above the surface of the Earth and the planetary and lunar orbits. The analogy functions also as a thought experiment, and Newton sketched a visual representation (figure 5.1) of the imagined successive paths of the projectile from the mountain to the Earth, ending with the escape velocity where it would, too, orbit the Earth under the effect of centripetal force.

Recall, too, Maxwell's vortex–idle wheel representation (see figure 2.13). It is a visual representation of an analogical model accompanied by text for how to animate it imaginatively, thus simulating a range of future states. S2 also drew several visual representations of his analogical models

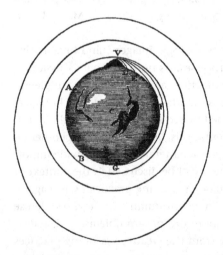

Figure 5.1
Newton's drawing of a projectile thrown from a high mountain with increasing velocity. *Principia*, vol. II, book III, 3.

and indicated simulating their motion through describing the motion, adding arrows to indicate motion and direction, and using gestures simulating motion (see, for instance, figures 3.4 and 3.14). The frequency of such instances in scientific thinking has led me to hypothesize that what is called "analogy" is often not neatly separable from imagistic and simulation processes as it customarily is in cognitive research.[1] Here again, considering cognition from the perspective of what scientists do can nudge cognitive science research in the direction of much needed integrative studies.

5.1 Model Construction and Analogy

There has been considerable interest in analogy in cognitive science in large part because it is a principal means through which people make inferences about novel experiences, phenomena, or situations, using what they already know and understand. It is, thus, central to understanding learning and problem solving and to developing expert computational systems. However, neither serious examination of how scientists use analogy nor mundane, spontaneous analogy use "in the wild" has contributed much to the development of the cognitive accounts. Our exemplars provide studies of self-generated, sophisticated, and reflective use of deep analogies. Both Maxwell and S2 had considerable knowledge of their source domains. Although we know nothing additional of S2 in this regard, Maxwell was a brilliant exploiter of analogy across the range of his work and highly reflective on his practice. There are some ways in which scientific analogizing practices do lie on a continuum with mundane cognitive practices, and we will consider these as the chapter unfolds. However, there are important ways in which the problem-solving episodes we have examined differ from those that have gone into current cognitive theories of analogy, most notably in that analogical sources do not provide ready-to-hand problem analogues from which a solution can be mapped and transferred. Instead, target and source domains interact through the construction of intermediate analog models and inferences about the source problem stem from these. Such differences lead to new ways of thinking about analogy.

The customary idea of problem solving by analogy is that one recognizes some similarities between the problem situation under consideration (target) and something with which one is familiar and is better understood (retrieval of source). One then creates a mapping between the two that enables solving the original problem (mapping and transfer). In the process, it is possible that the source and target need to be re-represented more abstractly in order for the comparison or mapping to be made. Take, for example, the solar system (source)—atom (target) analogy, usually attributed to Rutherford.[2] The sun and nucleus need to be represented more abstractly along the lines of "centrally located entities," and the planets and electrons as "entities that revolve around centrally located entities," in order to posit that similar forces are keeping the entities in orbit. This kind of re-representation is an instance of what I earlier called "abstraction via generic modeling." A "centrally located entity" is a generic representation of "sun-in-center" and of "nucleus-in-center." Once each phenomenon is understood in terms of the generic representation of "centrally located entities with entities revolving around them," one can reason about whether they actually do belong to the same class of phenomena by testing how inferences from one might apply to the other. Relevant dissimilarities can also be exploited, such as that electrons would lose energy while in orbit.

There are many instances of direct use of ready-to-hand analogical sources by scientists even in periods of conceptual change, such as Galileo's analogies between the moon and a wall made of stone that he used to cast doubt on the "perfect" nature of the heavenly bodies. What is extraordinary in Galileo's context is the very notion of making a comparison between a celestial object and an earthly one, but once one has the idea, the reasoning proceeds straightforwardly between the target (moon) and analogical source (wall) to produce inferences about what appear to be shadows, mountains, and craters on the moon. The striking feature about the use of analogical sources in our exemplars is that information from the source domain is not mapped directly to the target problem; rather the source domain provides information (constraints) that together with information (constraints) from the target domain is used to create intermediary hybrid models, possessing their own model constraints through which the problem solvers think and reason.[3] These imaginary models provide parallel worlds within which to reason about selected features—built into the models—of the real-world phenomena under investigation. Since the objective is to focus selectively on the relevant pieces, the models work well enough for reasoning purposes even though what is represented might not fully be feasible as real-world entities, processes, or situations. In each case the problem solution is an incremental process where a constructed model leads to target insights, which in turn lead to the construction of another model. When the problem is solved in the model, it, then, provides an analogical source from which to map a solution to the original (target) problem. My argument here is that analogy, as commonly understood, stands at one end of a continuum of "model-based reasoning." Examining the more complex cases where the analogical source model needs to be *constructed* will further insights into the nature of the creative reasoning that can be done with models, and into the nature of analogy itself.

How the models in our exemplars were constructed, manipulated, and modified has been addressed in detail in chapters 2 and 3. Here I provide a reminder summary. In deriving a mathematical representation for the field conception of forces, Maxwell constructed a series of hybrid electro-magnetic–mechanical models. The source domains of continuum mechanics and machine mechanics provided constraints that were fitted with constraints from the domain of electromagnetism to construct models that served as representations intermediary between the domains. The initial vortex model captured the geometric and kinematic constraints of various magnetic phenomena in producing the lines of force. However, this model was not sufficient for representing the interaction between electricity and magnetism because its mechanism would create jamming of the vortices due to friction among them. Recognizing this led Maxwell to call upon knowledge of gear mechanisms and to import dynamical relations between gears and idle wheels into a modified model that had the capacity to represent the causal structure of electromagnetic induction. Finally, the phenomena of electrostatic induction were captured by endowing the vortices with elasticity, which enabled calculating the propagation of forces within the model. At each phase of model construction Maxwell derived equations that were interpreted, through appropriate mappings, as representing the structure of various relations among parts of a model—first on the continuum-mechanical interpretation and then on the electromagnetic interpretation.

In the S2 case, the source (rod) and target (spring) domains were initially thought to be the same (the rod is just an unwound spring), but then a critical difference between them led S2 to realize a salient target constraint (the uniform distribution of the stretch of a spring) that then became operative for all subsequent model construction. That is, he inferred that the mechanism through which a rod bends is not of the same kind as that through which a spring stretches, and thus the bending rod model does not represent the spring's stretch. S2's knowledge of the behavior of rods and of geometrical and topological structures and transformations served as sources of constraints for building and transforming hybrid rod–spring models. He went through several iterations of constructing such models and simulating their stretching behaviors until he had created a model of the same kind with respect to the mechanism of stretch, and recognized that a twisting force (torsion) provides the explanation for the even distribution of the stretch of a spring.

To have a basis from which to compare the cognitive research on analogy with these exemplars, I focus on one reasoning segment of each: introducing idle wheels (Maxwell) and recognizing torsion (S2).

5.1.1 Introducing Idle Wheels

In this segment, Maxwell made an analogy in the service of modifying the model so as to use it in reasoning about electromagnetic induction. At the point where Maxwell recognized a major problem with his first model, he had already derived mathematical representations relating to various magnetic phenomena, such as magnetic induction and the dipolar nature of magnetism. In discussing this reasoning segment it will be helpful to repeat the visual representations of his models from chapter 2.

With continuum mechanics as a source domain, there was no ready-to-hand system in that domain from which to construct an analogy. Rather, Maxwell used constraints from the target domain to guide the selection of constraints from the source domain in constructing the initial vortex fluid model (figure 5.2a), which is a hybrid representation integrating those constraints (note: all the figures except (d) are my renderings from

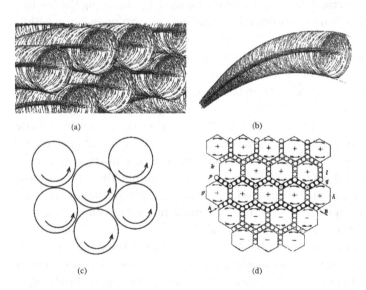

(a)   (b)

(c)   (d)

Figure 5.2
Visual representations of Maxwell's models.

Maxwell's descriptions). Thinking of electromagnetism as a continuum-mechanical system enabled Maxwell to draw on mathematical representations customarily applied in that domain. In the mathematical analysis of magnetic phenomena Maxwell needed only to consider the limiting case of one vortex (b). Once he derived a mathematical representation on the mechanical interpretation, Maxwell constructed several mappings between magnetic quantities and model quantities that he used throughout the entire analysis, such as that the magnetic intensity is related to the velocity gradient of the vortex at the surface. This mapping is possible because the model embeds electromagnetic constraints, as well as continuum-mechanical constraints. Further, it is possible to check that the derivations from it fit with other known mathematical representations such as the differential form of Ampère's law.

Whereas in deriving the equations for magnetic phenomena it was possible to ignore vortex interactions, to derive equations relating electricity and magnetism, such as electromagnetic induction, requires considering the entire vortex medium. This presents a problem, however: if the vortices are in motion, they touch one another and friction will create jamming. So, the initial model is not a feasible mechanical system. I have represented the problem schematically as a cross-section in figure 5.2c. My drawing of a cross-section is consistent with Maxwell's own use of cross-sectional drawings of vortices in his analysis. Next Maxwell made an analogy between the model (now acting as the target) and machine mechanics (source) in order to modify the initial model. The newly constructed hybrid model (fig. 5.2d) embeds constraints arising from all three domains. As we saw, Maxwell repeatedly stressed that this vortex–idle wheel model is to be understood itself as a representation of causal relations and not specific causal mechanisms. Figure 5.3 illustrates my account of the inferences likely to have led to the construction of the new model.

In this piece of reasoning, taking the initial model as the target, Maxwell's problem was to make the vortices interface in such a way that there would be no jamming. Referring to figure 5.3, on my interpretation, he first abstracted from the initial model a model of spinning wheels that touch (A). The abstract model of spinning wheels reminded him of specific mechanical systems containing machine gears (B), and he noticed an analogy between the vortices and machine gears (C). This gave him a source domain, but how the analogy might provide a new mode of connection for the vortices was not immediately evident. He thought about real-world gear connections that solved the jamming problem for machines (he mentioned several). From these he abstracted a model of idle wheel

Modes of Connection:

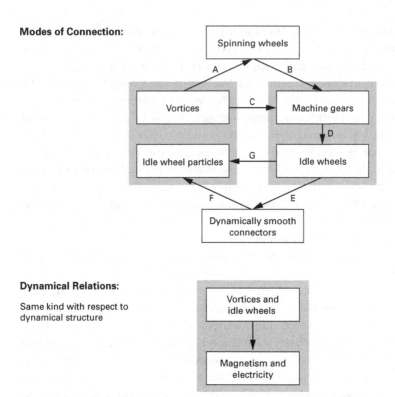

Dynamical Relations:

Same kind with respect to
dynamical structure

Figure 5.3
Introducing idle wheels.

connectors (D), and then further abstracted from that model to a model of a generic kind of connection, dynamically smooth connectors (E). Finally, he instantiated the dynamically smooth connectors in the form of what he dubbed "idle wheel particles" (F) between the vortices, thereby constructing the model represented by figure 5.2d.

It required further reasoning to "fit" the idle wheels to the model configuration smoothly. The specifics of the instantiation were guided by the mechanical constraints of the analogous case of idle wheels (G), the electrodynamic constraints of the target system, and specific constraints of the model. For instance, electromagnetic induction requires that the model idle wheels, unlike those in most real machines, have translational motion (needed for conducting media) and that heat is lost when in translational motion (the currents they represent loose heat). Considerations stemming from the interface between the particles and the vortices as represented in the model require the vortices to be treated as approximating rigid pseudospheres. Figure 5.2d is Maxwell's rendering of a cross-section of the three-dimensional vortex–idle wheel model. Presumably he drew the vortices as hexagons (his previous renderings were of circular cross sections) to convey the idea that the particles are tightly packed around them. Nothing hinges on this rendering of shape since in the limit their three-dimensional motion would satisfy the requisite topological constraints.

We can see then that although a concrete mechanism is provided, in reasoning by means of it, the vortex–idle wheel model (figure 5.2d) is taken to represent the *causal structure* of a class of dynamical systems. He was not positing that the phenomena of electromagnetic induction are actually created by the specific mechanism of vortices and idle wheels. The actual underlying causes in the aether were not known, and determining these was not the objective of this analysis. Rather, his contention was that the dynamical relations represented in the model between the idle wheel particles and vortices are of the same kind as the dynamical relations between electricity and magnetism in the process of induction. So, deriving mathematical equations for the model phenomena that capture the causal relational structures would provide equations for the macroscopic phenomena of electromagnetic induction under suitable mappings. For instance, since the equation for the flux density of the particles has the same form as the Ampère equation for closed circuits, it can be taken to represent the electric current density.

The point of how to understand the relation between the model and the phenomena is driven home when we take into account that for Maxwell electrical charge was not associated with particles, as on the modern view, but with tension or stress in the aetherial medium (as on Faraday's view). Thus Maxwell did not hypothesize that current is actually the flow of particles, but only that the causal relations between the idle wheels and vortices capture the causal relations between electricity and magnetism in induction. I have worked out several of Maxwell's mappings in section 2.2.2.

5.1.2 Recognizing Torsion

In this segment, S2 constructed a new kind of model—one that is three-dimensional—that allowed him to simulate the interaction between bending and stretching, and the novel insight deriving from this model was used to solve the target problem. We begin at the point where S2 constructed a model that enabled him to recognize the contribution of the force of torsion to the uniform distribution of a spring's stretch. He had just been considering a limiting case of a spring: a three-dimensional circle

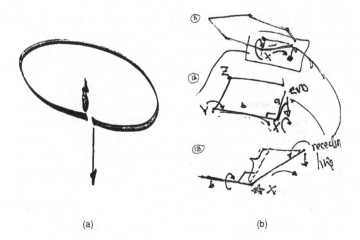

(a)   (b)

Figure 5.4
S2's three-dimensional circular coil and polygonal coil drawings.

with a break in it such that a downward force could be applied to it (figure 5.4a). In discussing this segment it will be helpful to repeat some of his drawings so we can refer to them.

One significant difference between this representation and his previous drawings of models is that it is three-dimensional, whereas his previous models were two-dimensional figures that could not represent twisting while stretching or bending. However, he did not immediately see the twist in the circular coil representation (figure 5.4a; see discussion of Model 4 in section 3.3.4). Rather, he began first to think about transmitting the force "from increment to increment of the spring." Segmenting the spring coil in this fashion led him to recall an earlier idea of a square spring which in the limit is "sort of like a circle." Thinking about a square figure, that is, one with side segments, led back to the original rod model, Model 1 (discussed in 3.4.1), and to imagining bending it up into a "series of approximations to the circle" (coil with side segments), thereby creating a series of polygonal coil models (figure 5.4b, 11–13) that are hybrid rod–springs. Here, too, the hexagonal and square springs are imaginary objects—not ones that S2 was thinking of as real springs, but as possibly capturing the dynamical relational structure between bending and stretching in a spring. He recognized that when a force is applied at the end of the open segment, there is a twist at the joint and *"you get a torsion effect"* in the adjacent segment. My interpretation of S2's inferences is represented schematically in figure 5.5.

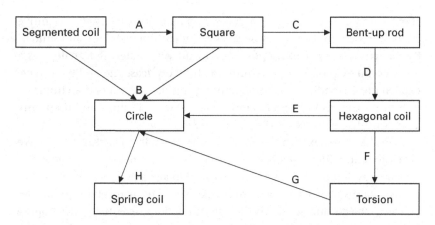

Figure 5.5
Inferring torsion.

Referring to figure 5.5, in thinking about segmenting the spring coil, S2 was reminded of an earlier idea of a square coil (A) that he did not pursue at the time he first thought of it. In the present context, he inferred that squares are like circles (B) when thought of in the limit of the segments of a coil, that is, in the case that these are infinitesimally small. This led him to consider bending up the rod so that it too was a segmented spring coil (C). Recall that the overarching problem for S2 at this point was determining the nature of the mechanism that makes for the difference between the way a rod bends and a spring stretches. The bent-up rod model is a hybrid of the two, in three-dimensions and oriented in the horizontal plane so as to enable imagining one's pulling down on the end of a segment as with the circular coil. He selected a specific rod–spring model, a hexagonal coil (D), and again assured himself that polygons—and specifically hexagons—are approximations to circles (E). He saw the effect of torsion in the hexagonal coil (F) and, carrying this information through an extrapolation of the hexagon to a circle once again (G), inferred that "maybe the behavior of the spring has something to do with the twist forces" (H). This latter reasoning served to eliminate the possibility that the fact that polygonal figures have joints is a significant difference between the polygonal coil models and a spring.

5.1.3 Experimental Research on Analogy
In the psychological literature, analogy is studied as a principal means by which people use what they know and understand to make inferences

about novel phenomena, experiences, or situations. Clearly the cognitive ability is rooted in the biological capacity for pattern matching and similarity recognition, most likely possessed by all vertebrates. But analogy is a more complex process that requires at the very least the ability to have explicit understanding of relations among objects, and, other than humans, only chimpanzees have been shown to be able to do this—and then only after considerable training (Premack 1983).

There has been extensive research on analogy in the area of cognitive development, which establishes that facility with analogy undergoes significant development from infancy to around age five. Analogy use begins as the infant's ability to make predictions based on perceptual similarities between objects and sensitivity to causal relations, eventually developing into a child's having the ability to engage fully in analogical problem solving (Carey 1985; DeLoache 1987; Gentner and Ratterman 1991; Gentner and Toupin 1986; Goswami 1992; Gosawmi and Brown 1989; Holyoak, Junn, and Billman 1984; Spelke 1991). Specifically, the five-year-old child typically displays the ability to recognize that the relationships in a known situation (source) can be used to make candidate inferences about an unknown (target).

There are several ways in which our exemplars accord with the cognitive science literature, but there are also important respects in which they contribute novel insights into analogical processes. One highly significant difference which has already been noted is that, unlike the experimental studies on which the cognitive theories of analogy are based, ready-to-hand analogical problem solutions are not transferred directly from the source to the target problem. In both exemplars, analogical domains serve as sources of constraints for use in constructing hybrid models. The problem solution is reached through investigating the interactions of constraints stemming from target, sources, and constructed models. Both exemplars make use of abstractive, simulative, adaptive, and evaluative reasoning in constructing a series of models. After each model is constructed, the dynamical behaviors of the model are determined, and then the model is evaluated as to whether it fits dimensions of interest in the target. In each case inferences are made from reasoning with the model and transferred to and evaluated with respect to the initial target, with goals and interpretations in guiding roles. Thus, a hybrid model, itself constructed on the basis of an analogy, serves as the basis of comparison with the target and provides the basis for problem solutions to be used in analogical inferences. In the retrieval, abstraction, construction, mapping, transfer, evaluation, and adaptation processes, subgoals and interpretations generated along the way determine which parts of a source analogy to use. This is so both when the source domains are used to create models and when potential solutions are mapped from the constructed models to the target phenomena. Although neither was expert in their problem domains, both Maxwell and S2 drew from source domains in which they had considerable expertise and experience in problem solving. Each represented the target problem with an emphasis on relational structures from the outset, and this representation guided the selection of the source domains. Their behavior corresponds to well-established findings that experts tend to focus on abstract relational information in problem solving, whereas novices tend to focus on surface similarities (Blanchette and Dunbar 2000; Chi, Feltovich and Glaser 1981; Clement 1986; Gentner and Ratterman 1991; Keane 1985 Novick 1988; Ross 1989).

Analogical processes of retrieval and of mapping and transfer have received considerable attention in the psychological literature. I consider these in turn.

5.1.3.1 Retrieval Despite the fact that people can recognize, comprehend, and use analogy, one consistent finding across the experimental literature is that retrieving an analogical source is difficult. This finding is to some extent likely an artifact of the way analogy use is studied in psychological experiments. Take, as an example, the "fortress–tumor" analogy problem, which might be considered the *C. elegans* of analogy research. That is, it plays the role of the paradigmatic "model organism" with which psychologists have conducted experiments on analogy.[4] The research line begun by Mary Gick and Keith Holyoak (1980) takes as its start the radiation problem of the Gestalt psychologist Kurt Duncker (1945), who used it as an ill-defined insight problem that people were asked to solve without being given a prior analogy. Gick and Holyoak developed their fortress analogy from two of the categories within which Duncker classified proposed solutions to the radiation problem: reducing the intensity of the rays as they pass through healthy tissue, and avoiding contact between the rays and healthy tissue (Gick and Holyoak 1980, 308).

In basic studies of analogical problem solving, participants (often undergraduates in introductory psychology classes) are given a story to read, such as the fortress story, and are told only that they are taking part in a comprehension study. Distracting stories are provided, and then the students are given a problem to solve, in this case the tumor problem, to see if they solve it by making an analogy with the fortress story. Surprisingly few participants spontaneously make the analogy between the source they

Fortress Story   A small country fell under the iron rule of a dictator. The dictator ruled the country from a strong fortress. The fortress was situated in the middle of the country, surrounded by farms and villages. Many roads radiated outward from the fortress like spokes on a wheel. A great general arose who raised a large army at the border and vowed to capture the fortress and free the country of the dictator. The general knew that if his entire army could attack the fortress at once it could be captured. His troops were poised at the head of one of the roads leading to the fortress. The ruthless dictator had planted mines on each of the roads. The mines were set so that small bodies of men could pass over them safely, since the dictator needed to be able to move troops and workers to and from the fortress. However, any large force would detonate the mines. Not only would this blow up the road and render it impassable, but the dictator would destroy many villages in retaliation. A full-scale direct attack on the fortress therefore appeared impossible.

The general, however, was undaunted. He divided his army up into small groups and dispatched each group to the head of a different road. When all was ready he gave the signal, and each group charged down a different road. All of the small groups passed safely over the mines, and the army then attacked the fortress in full strength. In this way, the general was able to capture the fortress and overthrow the dictator.

Tumor Problem   Suppose you are a doctor with a patient who had a malignant tumor in his stomach. It is impossible to operate on the patient, but unless the tumor is destroyed the patient will die. There is a kind of ray that can be used to destroy the tumor. If the rays reach the tumor all at once at a sufficiently high intensity, the tumor will be destroyed. Unfortunately, at this intensity the healthy tissues that the rays pass through on the way to the tumor will also be destroyed. At lower intensities the rays are harmless to healthy tissue, but they will not affect the tumor either. What type of procedure might be used to destroy the tumor with the rays and at the same time avoid destroying the healthy tissue?

Figure 5.6
Initial formulation of the fortress–tumor analogy pair (Gick and Holyoak 1980, 307–308, 351).

have just read and the problem; consistently across studies, nearly eighty percent failed. Once given the hint to use the fortress story, however, nearly seventy percent were able to solve the tumor problem using the fortress analogy. These findings replicate across different story pairs bearing the same relational structures in a wide range of analogy research. All kinds of experimental manipulations have been done to create variants of the experiment, such as telling the students to sketch the stories as they read or giving them visual formulations of the source story. I will discuss some of the successful manipulations in later sections.

In numerous other studies of retrieval and mapping behavior, nonexpert retrieval at all ages is strongly correlated with shared surface similarities (Keane 1985; Kolodner 1993; Ross 1989). Thus, one major stumbling block is thought to be the significant dissimilarities in surface features of the target and source, such as between soldiers and rays (lasers in some versions) and between capturing a fortress and destroying a tumor. In all likelihood, participants do not create more abstract representations of these stories as they read them in the course of the experiment. In our exemplars, although no direct analogies exist, unlike the experimental studies, retrieval of the source domains and the requisite constraints to make use of them seems not difficult. The scientists are drawing on deep understanding of the source domains and representational practices of their communities, and resorting to analogy seems a natural course to solving the problems. Kevin Dunbar has also noted the ease of analogy retrieval and use "in the wild," both in his studies of scientists and in more ordinary problem solving, such as political arguments (Dunbar and Blanchette 2001). When people make spontaneous analogies in meaningful problem-solving contexts, they draw on things with which they are familiar, whereas the psychological experiments require them to recall and use what they have just learned to solve problems that are not their own.

One finding deriving from the fortress–tumor experiments (which is also replicated in other studies) is that when participants are required to do some work in analyzing or comparing analog models, or to solve several analog problems, they frequently abstract a relational "schema" that they then use more easily in future problems (Gick and Holyoak 1983; Faries and Reiser 1988; Schumacher and Gentner 1988). This finding, too, corresponds with our exemplars. S2 can be interpreted as using topological schemas in making transformations of the models, and, given that he took Ph.D. qualifying exams in topology, we can assume that these derive from his having done significant problem solving. Maxwell drew abstract relational structures from continuum mechanical domains in which he previously had done significant mathematical analyses, and during the course of problem solving, he abstracted a schema of general dynamical relations pertaining to electromagnetism that he used in later problem solving in that area. That schema, which comprises relations common to both the target (electromagnetism) and the source (mechanics), represents what he called a "connected system." That he abstracted this general dynamical schema in the course of his problem solving and used it productively in the 1864 analysis lends support to my argument in chapter 2. Maxwell, contrary to what is claimed in some of the philosophical and historical analyses of his work, did not know how to apply general dynamics directly to electromagnetism until he had done the work of abstracting generic representations for velocity, momentum, and kinetic and potential energy from the constructed models (see, especially, figure 2.18).

In both of our exemplars, inferences, including erroneous inferences, can be traced directly to the constructed models, as is the case with empirical investigations of reasoning with analogies that serve as mental models for a domain (Gentner and Gentner 1983; Kempton 1986). Indeed, interpreting Maxwell as reasoning through the constructed models gives a better fit with the historical data in that there is no need to discount inconvenient pieces such as his "errors" in sign. What others have interpreted as errors are not mistakes once we construe Maxwell as reasoning through the models that are in play at those parts of the analysis. For instance, we saw that the negative sign in the equation he derived for the displacement current is correct if Maxwell is understood as reasoning through the model of an elastic medium: the restoring forces *should* be oriented in the opposite direction to the imposed force. Further, features of the models led directly to novel inferences about the target domain such as that the velocity of propagation in the model is the same as for the speed of light, and thus possibly for electromagnetic wave propagation, even though this had not yet been observed experimentally. There is further evidence of Maxwell's thinking through the constructed models in that traces of features of those models remained in future derivations throughout the rest of his work on electromagnetism (Nersessian 1984a, 2002c).

5.1.3.2 Mapping and Transfer Much of the cognitive science literature on analogy has focused on processes of mapping and transfer. Leaving aside for the moment that analogies are not mapped directly from source domains to targets in the exemplars, wherever mapping and transfer do take place, these largely involve making use of relational structures, as is consistent with the cognitive literature. In these processes, both exemplars fit the criteria for what makes an analogy productive proposed by psychologist Dedre Gentner. Her "structure mapping" criteria (which are widely agreed on in cognitive science) are: (1) structural focus (preserving relational structures); (2) structural consistency (making isomorphic mappings between systems); and (3) systematicity (mapping systems of higher-order, interconnected relational structures) (Gentner 1983; Clement and Gentner 1991; Gentner, Ratterman, and Forbus 1993).

There are two features of Gentner's criteria that make significant contributions to understanding analogical reasoning. First, the focus she places on mapping relational structures is especially important for understanding the productivity of these practices in science.[5] Analogical reasoning cannot be evaluated as "sound" in the logical sense, where true premises and good reasoning lead to true conclusions. But there are ways of differentiating instances of good analogical reasoning from less useful or bad. Gentner's criteria provide a means for evaluating the "goodness" of an analogy, that is, for determining *what* makes a particular analogy productive when it has proven fruitful and for thinking about *how* to make productive analogies (Gentner, Ratterman, and Forbus 1993).

Second, Gentner's systematicity criterion is a novel and valuable insight. It is not mapping of relational structures alone, but mapping of interconnected systems of such structures—that is, maintaining higher-order relations—that tends to make analogies most productive. Accessing a systematic representation of knowledge in the source domain provides a series of interconnected inferences to apply to the target or, as in our cases, to apply in model construction. In the fortress–tumor problem, for example, mapping of the interconnected relational structure "dividing the army avoids the mines and causes the capture of the fortress" leads to the inference that distributing the rays will avoid tissue damage and cause the death of the tumor. For Maxwell, mapping systems of causal relations enabled him to use the representational capacities of the mathematics that was being applied successfully to continuum phenomena such as fluids and elastic solids (what later became known as partial differential equations and vector analysis). For S2, thinking about interconnected relations between structure and behavior led to using representational resources of geometry and topology to connect the rod and spring models.

However, how Maxwell and S2 arrived at what to map and transfer diverges from Gentner's purely syntactic theory of structural alignment and projection. On her theory, the structures of relational matches are transferred as identities (even if some re-representation is required to achieve this) and candidate inferences are made on the basis of systematicity in the source domain. Her account, thus, assumes that goals and semantic information are not involved in mapping and transfer. Gentner, Kenneth Forbus, and other colleagues argue that a general theory of analogy as a cognitive capacity needs to capture all forms, including literary comparisons, proportional analogies, problem solving, and reasoning. They hold that this objective requires a purely syntactic theory of mapping and transfer since, for instance, people can process analogies without any goals, such as when a person understands an analogy they simply hear or read (Forbus et al. 1998). The core of an analogy does lie in a relational comparison, but which relations are to be compared and how are they selected? Keith Holyoak and Paul Thagard argue that, at the very least, transfer requires evaluating the plausibility of an inference in the context, and thus semantic and pragmatic information help to determine the candidate mappings and what to transfer, and, indeed, are operative in all of the processes of analogy (see Holyoak and Thagard 1996 for a succinct summary).[6] They base their claim on extensive psychological studies by Holyoak and studies of scientific analogies by Thagard. We can see that their "multiconstraint theory" better fits mapping and transfer processes in our cases with a few examples.

Maxwell's initial representation of his problem, for instance, includes the goal of finding a "continuous-action" representation for electromagnetic phenomena starting from specific constraints derived from that domain. He made explicit use of the goal and initial target constraints— and his representations of the target and source are informed by the question of what kind of continuum mechanical system will satisfy these constraints. Further, the interpretation of the models as continuum mechanical systems guides the selection of what mappings are relevant. S2's elaborated representation of the problem includes the goal of finding the mechanism through which springs stretch. The initial constraints are clearly delineated in the statement of the problem, and the additional constraint that the slope of the stretching spring remains constant was arrived at in the first few minutes of his reasoning. That is, the *dis*analogy between rod and spring led him to re-represent the target to include the uniform stretch of the spring. This revised goal and problem interpretation inform what behaviors of constructed models he focused on in mapping inferences.

The general pattern of the exemplars is that the interpretation of the target constraints and the goals of the target problem guide the selection of the salient constraints and candidates for transfer within the source domains. These, in turn, provide additional constraints on constructing models through which the problem solver reasoned about the phenomena in question. What mapping is made between the model and the target and what inferences transfer is guided by the interpretation and goal in play at the particular stage of problem solving. The representation-building aspect of analogy as evidenced in the exemplars points to significant processes that are missing in investigations of analogy in the cognitive science literature.

5.1.4 Representation Building

Looking at the cognitive science literature, then, we find two places where what is investigated as analogy enters into our exemplars: first, in the selection of a source domain from which to draw constraints for model construction; and second, whenever features of a constructed model are mapped to the target phenomena. The kind of creative work evidenced in *building the model representations* that are central to understanding how the analogies function to solve their respective problems is not addressed.[7]

Our exemplars illustrate what is a common practice across the sciences. In tackling complex, ill-defined problems scientists often create models through which to reason about the target phenomena. In cases where little is known about the target, analogy can provide a means of building the model, through the kinds of constraint-satisfaction processes we have been considering. The way in which the model is constructed determines the nature of the analogical comparison between target, source, and model objects, entities, or processes. Constraints of the target problem determine which constraints of the source domain are potentially relevant, and these are incorporated into a model related to both domains. The warrant one has for believing that reasoning with the model can reveal understanding about the target stems from how it is constructed. For instance, S2's hexagonal spring model affords a comparison between its behavior and that of a real-world spring because the model was constructed to be related to the spring in ways germane to the target problem. The model object has a configuration that is understood to be related to the circular shape of the spring in specific ways and an orientation related to the stretch of a spring when pulled downward. Thus, after imagining its stretch led to the insight of torsion, which satisfies also the target constraint of uniform stretch, S2 was warranted in transferring that causal mechanism to the spring and pursuing the implications.

Likewise, to understand the nature of the comparison between the analogical domains of continuum mechanics and machine mechanics and the target domain of electromagnetism, one needs to address how the intermediary model representations were constructed. Beyond the initial, rudimentary comparison, the comparison is *indirect*, stemming from the interaction of target and source constraints in the models. When mathematical representations were derived for a hybrid model, the nature of its construction dictated how they were to be mapped to the initial target. In this way, solving model problems can provide candidate solutions to target problems. In the segment of reasoning outlined in section 5.1.1, Maxwell was led to a way of representing the dynamical relations involved in electromagnetic induction by means of vortex–idle wheel interactions through solving a problem that arises in the vortex model (friction). In the segment of reasoning outlined in section 5.1.2, S2 was led to a way of representing the mechanism of the uniform stretch of a spring by means of the twist in the stretch of a polygonal coil through solving a problem that arises in the rod models ("drooping"). The processes of construction led to models in which the novel features emerged. Insights resulting from the hybrid melds were explored, in conjunction with physical realizations such as drawings and gestures, and through expression in other representational formats, such as mathematics and language.

The exemplars provide a significant contrast that underscores that although structure mapping provides criteria for evaluating the goodness of a mapping, it is not sufficient to explain how mappings are determined. The interpretation in the problem solving context determines what model relations one is warranted in transferring. Once S2 understood that torsion determines the stretch of the polygonal springs, he transferred this causal mechanism to the stretch of a spring. He had good reasons for doing so because of his understanding that the polygonal coils approximate a circle as the sides become increasingly smaller. Maxwell, on the other hand, did not transfer the causal mechanism of vortex–idle wheel motion to the electromagnetic aether; there were no electromagnetic grounds for that inference. Indeed, the specific mechanism was quite implausible even for motion in a continuum-mechanical system. That mechanism derived from an analogy between the model and machine mechanics. It solved the problem of friction in the model, and because it was interpreted as representing a generic causal structure (a "connected system"), it solved the problem of representing electromagnetic induction. In sum, it would be impossible to make sense of how the relational comparisons get made in these cases if we considered only retrieval, mapping, and transfer, and omitted the processes involved in building the model representations.

Finally, to understand how the sources contributed to conceptual change also requires considering the nature of the iterative model-building processes in bootstrapping. The hybrid models afford exploring novel *combinations* of constraints—not represented in either target or source domain. It is conceivable that one iteration could be sufficient, but conceptual change in science is difficult. It is more plausible that the incremental processes displayed in the exemplars are the norm. Radical reconceptualization of a domain is likely to require more than just constructing a single, well-articulated model; it more likely requires a series of models that serve as building blocks, moving increasingly far from the starting point until reaching the problem solution, and thus creating the conceptual changes.

Looking at the science end of the spectrum of complexity in problem solving using analogy calls to the fore the importance of building the representation for mapping after retrieval in mundane cases as well. With the fortress–tumor problem, for instance, the problem solver would need to build a representation such that dividing an army to capture the fortress and using a number of rays of lesser intensity to kill the tumor will match in an isomorphic mapping. This might be an easier task than the representation building in our exemplars; nevertheless, the reasoning involved is not trivial. There is no reason to assume, for instance, that people have ready to hand some abstract representation of "intensity" that readily connects it to a matching representation of "divide." Indeed reexamining existing data in the literature with respect to the question of whether and how intermediate representations are created might lead to a reinterpretation of the reasoning processes.

Even in mundane cases, retrieval, mapping, and transfer are likely to be much more cognitively complex phenomena than is usually assumed. Retrieval of a source can indeed occur in a flash of insight, but then the hard intellectual work of how to exploit it begins. I suspect the reason why representation-building processes have not received as much attention as other processes is that in the psychological experiments the analogy that will solve the problem is most often provided in advance. The objective is to get the person to retrieve it and ideally use it correctly (mapping and transfer as the experimenter has designed). Casting the net wider to include self-generated analogies in problem solving, especially in science, however, reveals the need for more empirical studies aimed at understanding a range of representation-building processes. Although our cases might be considered extraordinarily creative, my intuition is that if spontaneous use of analogy—in protocol experiments or "in the wild"—were to be investigated systematically, building intermediary hybrid mental models would be seen to be a significant dimension of mundane usage. In sum, analogy comprises many processes, and the focus of current research leaves much of what is creative about such reasoning unaccounted for.

5.1.5 Exemplification

Attending to representation building in analogy points to another consideration absent from the analogy literature. Specifically, what enables the reasoner to have some assurance that he or she is on a productive path using a particular analogical representation (constructed or retrieved) and that the model solution is likely to be applicable to the target problem? This problem leaps to the fore in our cases because the problem solutions are transferred from imaginary models, so why would anyone think they could provide solutions to real-world problems? That is, the analogical comparisons are built on imaginative, "what if" reasoning; the models are not true or false representations of the phenomena. The hybrid model is an object of thought in its own right, constructed to provide a relational comparison with the phenomena of interest.

Inferences made from a model can, of course, be formulated as propositions that are true or false—"electric and magnetic forces are propagated at the speed of light"—but their truth or falsity is not determined on the basis of the comparison alone. The most reasoning from the model can do is provide inferences about targets that are warranted to pursue. From what does the warrant derive? Even if the "structure mapping" criteria provide conditions necessary for a productive analogy, they are not sufficient to account for how it is that reasoning through a relational comparison between a model and a target is a reliable strategy for making inferences about the specific phenomena under investigation. Attending to the representation-building processes provides significant clues.

In the philosophical literature on models, several accounts propose that "similarity" is the basis of the representational relation between a model and the real-world phenomena. A widespread complaint about similarity accounts of representation charges, correctly, that nearly anything is similar to anything else when viewed in the right way (see, e.g., Goodman 1968). Ronald Giere adds the qualifier that models are similar to what they represent to "a specified set of respects and degrees" (Giere 1988, 93). Although respects could be specified as those that are "relevant," what would constitute an adequate metric for "degrees" is unclear. I argued in earlier work that the "same kind" criterion indicates that "isomorphism," rather than just "similarity," is the basis of productive model-based reasoning in science. I now agree with the critique that although isomorphism narrows the notion of degrees, isomorphic matching structures can be accidental as well (Suarez 2003). Also, although isomorphism is a desideratum in the scientific cases, it is too stringent a criterion for all cases of productive analogy (Holland et al. 1986). I did maintain that the models need to be isomorphic to relevant respects of the phenomena they model. The issue is that not just any isomorphism is relevant. Neither will just any set of matching structural relations do; so Gentner's systematicity criterion works only to narrow the scope of candidate inferences. To attain the epistemic goals of reasoning through models requires that an analogical match to the target problem be selective in the relevant ways with respect to the problem at hand.

We have seen repeatedly that the overarching criterion for evaluating whether a constructed model was satisfactory in our cases required the model to be of the "same kind" as the target phenomena along particular dimensions. The notion that selected model structures *exemplify* the phenomena under investigation serves to explicate the "same kind" criterion, and assists understanding how reasoning by means of a model leads to reliable inferences about the phenomena.[8] As introduced by Nelson Goodman in *Languages of Art* (Goodman 1968), a representation exemplifies certain features or properties if it "both is and refers to" something which has those features or properties; that is, "[e]xemplification is possession plus reference" (1968, 53). One of his examples is that of a tailor's fabric swatch, which "is a sample of color, weave, texture, and pattern; but not of size, shape, or absolute weight or value" (ibid.).

Goodman's notion readily applies to certain kinds of physical models such as those of vascular processes that biomedical engineers use in performing simulations (Nersessian and Patton, in press). I recognize that using exemplification to apply to conceptual models might strike some readers as odd. After all, Goodman's examples are of real objects that have the properties in question, whereas the models I am talking about are imaginary. I think the notion can be extended productively to comprise abstractions, such as the notion that the model both refers to and has the "causal relational structure" of electromagnetic phenomena in the Maxwell case or the "causal relation of torque to stretch" of a spring in the S2 case. It helps to underscore that the models are constructed such that the isomorphism between the relational structure in the model and the phenomena is not arbitrary, but actually *is* the relational structure in question.

Catherine Elgin (Elgin 1996, in press) has built on Goodman's notion to address the epistemic problem that science makes extensive use of practices that, if we insist on equating truth and epistemic acceptability, lead clearly to falsehoods, such as limiting case demonstrations, idealizations, curve smoothing, and computational simulations. Yet science accepts the outcomes of such practices as advancing scientific goals, which include deriving a mathematical representation through idealization or predicting future states on the basis of a computational simulation. One can infer from this either that science is cognitively defective or allow that scientific understanding "is often couched in and conveyed by symbols that are not and do not purport to be true" (Elgin 2004, 116). Elgin advocates that the epistemic value of modeling, as well as other strategies and symbols used by scientists, lies in their ability to exemplify, that is, to "at once refer to and instantiate a feature" even if that feature is an abstraction (Elgin 1996, 171). As she points out, physical exemplifications are routinely created for experimental purposes such as when a lump of ore is refined to consist only of iron. Such physical abstractions enable the solving of problems that pertain to the specific properties of iron in the context of experimentation. Applied to conceptual models, the notion of exemplification captures the idea of selective representation—that is, that a model needs to capture the abstract features along the relevant dimensions given specific goals and purposes. Note that our case studies themselves are exemplifications in the context of this book: They both have and refer to the features of model-based reasoning in conceptual change that I wish to examine.

The representation-building practices of both S2 and Maxwell can be understood as seeking to understand the target phenomena through constructing models that exemplify selective features under investigation in the target domain. In the relational comparisons between a model and what it represents, it is those structures in the model that exemplify the relevant features (are of the "same kind as") of the target phenomena that have the potential to yield understanding of the phenomena. One can, then, conduct manipulations of models in place of manipulating the phenomena, and come to understand something about the phenomena. Maxwell's vortex–idle wheel model, for example, exemplifies the causal relational structure of electric and magnetic interactions in inductive phenomena. Reasoning about the causal relations between vortices and idle wheels informs him about how to mathematically represent the causal relations of electromagnetic induction. S2's hexagonal spring model exemplifies the causal relationship between twisting and stretching in a spring. Reasoning about the causal relations in the model informs him about the effects of torsion in the spring.

Constructing a conceptual exemplification of abstract relational structures is the mental equivalent of the purified iron exemplar. Given the way the model is constructed in the S2 case, the imagined action of stretching a polygonal coil simultaneously instantiates "a twist force while stretching" (a kind of simulation the rod model does not afford) and refers to "a twist force while stretching" in the comparison object, the spring. Since the twist would keep the stretch of the polygonal coil uniform, these models provide appropriate comparisons to the germane feature of the spring whereas the rod models do not. So, S2 could be reasonably secure in transferring the inference that torsion controls stretching in the model case to the case of the spring. In the Maxwell case, once he had assured himself that, under the appropriate interpretations, the causal relations between the vortices and idle wheels that allow motion in the medium do exemplify the causal relations between electricity and magnetism in induction, he could be reasonably secure in transferring the general dynamical mathematical representation he derived for the model to electromagnetism.

Selectively constructing the models so as to satisfy constraints deemed germane enables the reasoner to bracket irrelevant (or potentially irrelevant) features, and serves to fix attention on those features relevant to the problem-solving context. *A satisfactory model is one that exemplifies features relevant to the epistemic goals of the problem solver.* Through the models the reasoner is able to grasp insights and gain understanding, and is warranted in pursuing where the inferential outcomes deriving from the model might lead with regard to the target phenomena. The same holds for my use of the S2 and Maxwell cases as exemplars. My strategy is not to try to generalize from cases, but to transfer insight and understanding from these exemplars to this kind of reasoning where it occurs across the sciences.

Finally, drawing on the notion of exemplification to explicate how constructed models are selective also serves as a reminder of the deeply sociocultural nature of representation.[9] As Goodman observed, more than one instantiation or realization of a model as an exemplification is possible, and the same model can be interpreted to exemplify different things, depending on one's goals, purposes, and context. For instance, a paint chip usually exemplifies a color, but it might in certain circumstances be taken to exemplify a geometrical shape, such as a rectangle. It exemplifies color within a particular set of social norms surrounding the practice of picking paint for one's walls or house. In their model-based reasoning practices, both Maxwell and S2 are drawing on a repertoire of representational practices and the conventions of specific communities surrounding these.

Investigating the processes of creating, manipulating, and adapting models in analogical reasoning points to yet another way our exemplars differ from analogy as studied in the cognitive science literature: imagistic representations and simulative imagining are used together with analogical reasoning. In chapters 2 and 3 we saw that both Maxwell and S2 can be interpreted as using imagery and mental simulation in retrieving sources, and constructing and making inferences through the models. Although there is now widespread acknowledgment that visual representations can play a role in analogy, and some recognition that mental simulation/animation could also be involved, there is scant cognitive research on such phenomena in analogical processes.

5.2 Imagistic Representation

The exemplars provide ample evidence of the use of imagistic representations in reasoning processes. In each case, the problem solver created external schematic representations of his constructed models and used these as ways of examining and exploring facets of those models, to make predictions, to convey insights to others, and, for Maxwell, to derive mathematical results. These drawings provide abstract structured representations of the core elements of the mental models through which the domains are interpreted. In this section I will examine the significant cognitive functions these kinds of representations serve for the individual reasoner and for communicative processes. For example, S2 stated the need to "fix" his initial mental model of the bending rod by drawing it in several positions (figure 3.4). These external representations allowed him to represent "snapshots" of behaviors, which were used to support his inference that the rod would "droop" as it bent, something he had inferred from imagining the behavior of the rod just prior to stating the need to draw it. The drawings also allowed for comparison with snapshots of the behavior of a stretching spring, subsequently drawn (figure 3.5) and superimposed on the initial drawing. Such side-by-side comparison of specific behaviors is not likely to be possible in working memory. In many instances he gestured motions over the drawings or in the air as he reported imagining simulations. These gestures could serve either to assist the internal simulation or to convey it to the interviewer.

Beyond the functions they served in his own reasoning, the drawings also served communicative purposes as S2 attempted to convey his mental models to the interviewer, possibly evoking the construction of a parallel mental model by the interviewer. So, too, Maxwell's diagram of the vortex–idle wheel representation provided a fixed representation for his imagined solution to the problem of "conceiving of the vortices in a medium, side by side, revolving in the same direction" (1861–1862, 468) with which he could interact while deriving the various components of mathematical analysis, and through which he meaningfully could communicate his thoughts to others.[10] Further, the specific imaginary mechanism Maxwell hit upon is not something that anyone in his community would have encountered before, and therefore he could assume it would be difficult for others to comprehend if it were communicated only in language or mathematics. Maxwell's diagram has the potential to help his readers *construct* their own mental models through which to understand the hybrid mechanism and, specifically, to focus attention on the abstract mechanics of the causal relations between the vortices and idle wheels from which the mathematical inferences derive. Just as S2 did, Maxwell provided arrows and instructions to indicate how to imagine the motion created at points of interaction is transmitted throughout the model.

Although the literature on imagery in both cognitive science and science studies concentrates on the visual modality, quite likely representations in the format of the full range of sensory modalities can be utilized in model-based reasoning.[11] Galileo, for instance, conducted experiments in which he strung bells along the path of an object rolling down an inclined plane to discover if he could hear the changes in speed—through changes in frequency of pitch—that were too rapid to be seen. Archeologists have been known to use kinesthetic information in constructing analogical models (Shelley 1996). Surgeons report visualizing organ shapes and patterns while touching them during surgical manipulations and thinking about how to proceed (Gatti 2005; Reiner 2004). Recall that S2 at one point calls the kind of imagery he is experiencing "kinesthetic." From the context, and together with his elaboration of the remark as meaning the bigger spring is more "floppy" and his hand motions, we can interpret him as experiencing something like the feel of jiggling a spring (such as a "slinky") in his hand. The wider coils would have a looser feel, and this leads to the inference that the spring with wider coils would stretch farther. One would expect, then, as with visual imagery, that simulations deriving from imagery associated with other senses would conform to internalized constraints about the way things feel, smell, and taste, during perception. Given the paucity of empirical investigations of other modalities, I concentrate on the visual modality, construed widely enough to encompass S2's gestured drawings.

In addition to creating the external representations, S2 claimed to be experiencing mental images prior to the representations he sketched and he gestured simulations over the drawings or into the air in front of him.[12] The predominant cognitive science literature has been directed toward visual mental imagery and has provoked considerable discussion in what Michael Tye (1991) dubbed "the imagery debate." Much of this literature is concerned with debating whether the images that participate in experiences of "pictures in the mind's eye" are epiphenomena or a fundamental form of representation used in cognitive processing. Although there are interesting issues there, that debate is largely irrelevant to the problem I am addressing. The most pertinent question here concerns the roles that external visual representations play in reasoning with mental models. What is significant from the imagery literature, as we saw in chapter 4, is that certain kinds of mental transformational processes are possible with internal representations, that these conform to real-world physical constraints, and that studies from cognitive neuroscience provide ample evidence of activity in the visual and motor processing areas of the brain during imaginative thinking. Whether or not one is consciously aware of mental imagery, external visual representations can still serve to engage internal cognitive processes. Niels Bohr, for one, claimed not to be able to visualize, but in his early work he drew many sketches and made three-dimensional physical models relating to his conceptualization of the atom.[13]

As argued in chapter 4, that mental models used in reasoning processes contain perceptual information does not require the reasoner to experience mental pictures. As Barsalou and others have argued, if perceptual simulation is accompanied by conscious visual imagery, additional processing is likely to be involved. It might turn out that this processing contributes something significant to mental modeling, but if so, determining what and how requires empirical research yet to be carried out. The issues at the core of our concerns here are: (1) what kinds of intellectual work can be done using imagistic representations in reasoning and problem solving; and (2) how might these be different from what can be done using only propositional representations. Much that is germane to these issues is covered in my discussion of iconic, propositional, modal, and amodal representations in chapter 4. What I want to bring to the fore in the discussion of imagistic representation here is the notion introduced there of "internal–external representational coupling" in mental modeling processes. That is, the external representation and the internal model are best understood as forming a system in deriving inferences. The earlier discussion pointed to thinking in ideomotor research in support of the notion of "coupling" of cognitive mechanisms and external representations. Here I consider what external imagistic representations might contribute in scientific reasoning processes. In each exemplar, key insights arose in interaction between the reasoner's mental models and the schematic drawings they created. The cognitive science literature on diagrammatic representation provides insights for a start on answering this question.

5.2.1 Cognitive Research on Diagrammatic Representations

The visual representations that figure prominently in our exemplars are line drawings that are schematic or diagram-like representations. These diagrams are of the interpretations of phenomena under investigation in terms of imaginary models. There are many forms of visual representation in science, but diagrams are most like the sketches scientists make while reasoning and while communicating with one another. They are two-dimensional representations fixed in time, but can be annotated to indicate a dynamical interpretation. As communicative devices, diagrams can serve to facilitate construction of shared mental models within a community, which in science would be of use in transporting models out of the local milieu of their construction. On the account of mental modeling in chapter 4, a significant role for diagrams would be facilitating reasoning through interplay with mental models to which they have such correspondences. As such, diagrams are to be understood as components of reasoning processes. To be clear, I am not claiming that there need be any *resemblances* between the internal and external representations. What I am claiming is that there are *correspondences* between elements of the mental models, which are interpretations, and the diagrams, which are understood in terms of the models and whatever conventions the community has about such representations. Insofar as there are correspondences between elements of mental models and elements represented in diagrams, manipulating the components of a diagrammatic representation as one perceives it or acts on it can lead to corresponding transformations of the mental model (see also Greeno 1989).

Though the cognitive mechanisms of how diagrams and mental models interact are not yet known (Scaife and Rogers 1996), a wide range of empirical data supports the view that in making explicit, highlighting, or supplying structural and behavioral information, diagrammatic representations provide constraints and affordances for inferences in reasoning processes. Although the empirical literature has largely not studied situations of self-generated diagrams in creative reasoning, what diagrams contribute to reasoning, problem solving, and learning has been the subject of wide investigation. This literature provides some useful insights for thinking about their role in creative reasoning, which I will discuss first and then consider our exemplars in light of this research.

The 1987 paper by Simon and Larkin launched a veritable industry dedicated to the study of diagrams: journals, conferences, a list-server, and at least one society. I make no pretensions to being familiar with all of it, but once again have selectively sampled the literature for that which is pertinent to establishing roles for such visual representations in mental modeling processes. There is widespread agreement that diagrams are important cognitive resources for reasoning and problem solving and significant consensus on the functions of diagrammatic representations in these cognitive processes (see, e.g., Glasgow, Narayanan, and Chandrasekaran 1995; Hegarty 2004). Clearly diagrams can serve as external memory, but the literature goes beyond this observation to address the perceptual affordances of diagrams, their capacity for representing structure, their capacity for representing conceptual information (especially causality), and the role of expertise in interpreting and using diagrams.

A common finding across the diagrams research is that how well a diagram works in facilitating thinking depends on how well it is designed and whether a person has the requisite skills and knowledge to make use of it. The conclusions that Simon and Larkin (1987) reached in arguing for why "a picture is (sometimes) worth 10,000 words" have been borne out in many subsequent investigations. These include that diagrams aid significantly in organizing cognitive activity during problem solving through fixing attention on the salient aspects of the problem, enabling retrieval and storage of salient information, exhibiting salient constraints (such as structural and causal constraints) in appropriate colocation, and, in general, colocating information that needs to be integrated in reasoning. By providing an explicit and fixed representation of locality information, such as neighborhood relations, relative size, and intersections, they facilitate using perceptual inferencing mechanisms. This affords insights that might be difficult or impossible to attain with propositional representations even if they are "informationally equivalent." Additional research has established that diagrams support causal and functional inferences. Janice Gobert and John Clement (1999), for example, showed that participants who drew diagrams had a better understanding of causal and dynamic relations involved in plate tectonics than those who only wrote summaries of what they read in the textbook. These results suggest, as do the mental animation studies discussed earlier, that highlighting spatial configurations such as adjacency facilitates grasping relational structure. For instance, a diagram of a pulley system can be understood to represent the causal relations and sequences among various parts of the device (Hegarty 1992).

The feature that they are "plane structure[s] in which representing tokens are objects whose mutual spatial and graphical relations are interpreted directly as relations in the target structure" (Stenning and Lemon 2001, 36) provides an indication of why diagrammatic representations would be useful for both analogy and mental modeling: One can represent and highlight higher-order conceptual relations and their interconnections by means of the spatial configurations (Johnson-Laird 2002; Shimojima 2001; Stenning and Lemon 2001).

Diagrams, then, can be used to represent the core structure of an interpretation or the conceptualization of a domain. Peter Cheng and Herbert Simon (1995) showed how diagrams were used to represent complex conceptual relations in historical scientific discoveries by Galileo (quickest descent problem) and Huygens and Wren (law of conservation of momentum). Cheng and colleagues (Cheng 1999a,b; Cheng, Lowe, and Scaife 2001; Cheng and Simon 1995) call these kinds of representations "law encoding diagrams (LED)" since they "capture the important laws or relations of a domain in the structure of a diagram using geometrical, spatial, and topological constraints, such that a single instantiation of a diagram represents one instance of a phenomenon" (Cheng and Simon 1995, 2). They can also serve to integrate information from different domains. Graphical representations provide good examples of such integration.

In a series of experiments, Meredith Gattis and Keith Holyoak (1996) explored manipulations of graphs integrating conceptual relations such as between temperature and altitude. Graphs provide especially good examples of a major feature that distinguishes diagrams from other forms of visual representation: lawlike constraints establish the correspondences between the diagram and what is represented (Shimojima 2001). One such constraint is the "slope mapping constraint": the horizontal axis represents the independent variable, and the vertical axis, the dependent (Gattis and Holyoak 1996). Under this constraint, a steeper line corresponds to a faster rate of change in the dependent variable with respect to change in the independent variable, such as with a temperature and altitude graph. They showed that when graphs adhered to this constraint, the participants in their study were able easily to make perceptual inferences about the depicted relations, which they were unable to do with graphs exhibiting the same information but violating this constraint. The constraint allows the conceptual relations to be "read off" of the representation. This finding underscores that familiarity with the conventions of a representational form enhances cognitive usefulness. Additionally, participants were significantly better at making correct inferences when the graphs had more abstract correspondences to what was represented, highlighting relations, rather than when they had higher pictorial correspondence. This and other research on diagrams indicate that suppressing irrelevant information in creating the external representation also serves to enhance its cognitive usefulness in reasoning.

Another way diagrams function in problem solving is by scaffolding simulation using perceptual and motor processes (Barsalou 1999; Glenberg 1997a). Craig, Nersessian, and Catrambone (2002a,b) argued that the way a diagram is drawn affects not only what is perceptually simulated, but also how the resulting simulation can be transformed. As discussed in chapter 4, a long history of findings dating back to Cooper and Shepard's (1973) chronometric studies of mental rotation, supports the premise that simulations are transformed through motor activity. More recently, researchers have found that simulated transformations are motorically structured and constrained. The ease with which imagined body parts are mentally rotated, for instance, parallels the ease with which those parts can be rotated in actuality (Parsons 1987). In addition, concurrent motor activity consistent with simulated transformations of imagined objects tends to make those transformations faster and more accurate, whereas inconsistent activities produce interference (Wexler, Kosslyn, and Berthoz 1998). Generally speaking, simulated transformations appear to be constrained in ways that parallel the way the world is constrained. Insofar as contextual aspects of diagrams would help determine the physical properties of simulated objects (texture, mass, shape, etc.) and the context in which they are perceived (perspective, orientation, scale, etc.), those aspects act as transformational affordances, facilitating certain simulated transformations while inhibiting others.

Diagrammatic representations can be useful, however, only if a person is in a position to take advantage of their representational characteristics (Stenning and Lemon 2001; Stenning 2002; Hegarty 2004; Chandrasekaran 2005), that is, if they can be interpreted meaningfully. Just as the squiggles that make up the words and sentences on this page have to be interpreted, so too do the markings on a diagram. To be interpreted meaningfully, diagrammatic representations have to conform to the conventions of the community, and these are learned. As Stenning notes in his analysis of sentential representations and diagrams in logical reasoning, "[a]long with squiggles, a community is internalized" (2002, 3). As one would expect, psychological research shows that the ability to interpret a diagram depends on the richness of knowledge the person has of the domain (Tabachneck-Schijf, Leonardo, and Simon 1997) and how well integrated his or her conceptual understanding is (Koedinger and Anderson 1990), and is thus related to his or her level of expertise.

But even to the expert, not just any diagram is worth 10,000 words. It needs to be well constructed, and one way in which it can be is through exemplifying the ideas—in particular relations—it is meant to represent and convey. Exemplification is important for both communication through diagrammatic representations and self-generated representations used during reasoning processes. Take, for instance, the diagrams used in the experiments on gears by Schwartz and Black (1996b). They found that when presented with more jagged drawings of gears, rather than drawings of smooth circles, participants were more likely to mentally simulate rotation in solving the problem of how the motion is transmitted.The jaggedness better exemplifies the causal idea that one gear drives the other, and thus serves to evoke a transformational simulation of the mental model.

A possible explanation as to why the diagram that was provided by Gick and Holyoak (1983) in one variation of the experiments on the fortress–tumor analogy problem did not facilitate solving the problem is the fact that the arrows do not exemplify the highly salient notion of intensity building at the point of focus in the diagram, as illustrated in figure 5.7.

Recall that the solution to the source problem of capturing the fortress requires that the army divide into smaller units and reassemble at the fortress, which is exemplified by a diagram showing the large arrow divided into smaller arrows converging at a location. The source and target problems, however, are dissimilar in that the ray to be aimed at the tumor breaks down not into smaller rays, as the army breaks down into smaller columns, but rather into rays of less intensity. The converging arrows exemplify only spatial relations, whereas what is required is a representation of the notion that the intensity is weak at the areas surrounding the tumor site, but grows at the site. Thus, Beveridge and Parkins (1987) improved performance significantly by showing participants transparent colored strips arranged in the same pattern as the converging arrows, but which started out lightly colored at the ends and increased to darkly colored at the center. Similarly, when shown an animated version of

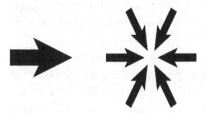

Figure 5.7
Convergence arrows similar to those used by Gick and Holyoak (1983) to help illustrate the events in the fortress story.

the converging arrows whose motion conveys the idea of increasing intensity, participants also performed significantly better (Pedone, Hummell, and Holyoak (2001). Craig, Nersessian, and Catrambone (2002a,b) showed that having people gesture the convergence through sliding wooden blocks and crashing them together also significantly increased the number of participants who solved the radiation problem. In these cases, it is not animation per se that facilitates solution, but that the animations (visual and motor) each exemplify that the intensity of force grows as convergence takes place. Used in conjunction with the fortress narrative they facilitate generating and simulating a mental model in which a growing intensity in force is represented and becomes a resource for solving the analogous radiation problem. That is, they activate a corresponding internal simulation.

Finally, the totality of the research on diagrams lends support to the contention that "external representations are not simply inputs or stimuli to the internal mind; rather they are so intrinsic to many cognitive tasks that they guide, constrain, and even determine cognitive behavior" (Zhang 1997, 180). There is ample evidence that active perception of diagrams while reasoning provides situational information to working memory that interacts with mental models and participates directly in reasoning. The internal and external representations are best understood as "coupled," each providing their own constraints and affordances, such that features of the external representations make direct contributions to transformations of the mental models and vice versa. Depending on how they are constructed they can facilitate or impede problem solving. In the studies of imagistic simulation that were discussed in chapter 4, generally speaking, simulated transformations appear to be constrained in ways parallel to how real interaction with the world is constrained. Insofar as contextual aspects of diagrams might help to determine the physical properties of simulated objects (such as texture, shape, mass) and the context in which they are perceived (such as perspective, orientation, scale), those aspects act as transformational affordances, facilitating certain simulated transformations while inhibiting others.

In our exemplars, the diagrammatic representations can be interpreted as indispensable components of reasoning processes that comprise internal and external representations of constructed models. Specifically, they act to facilitate imagining three-dimensional phenomena and processes taking place in time (see also Gooding 2005). To support this claim, I will walk through an extended segment of S2's reasoning, followed by a shorter segment of Maxwell's reasoning, drawing on the experimental findings.

5.2.2 Recognizing Torsion (Redux)

S2 drew all of his rod models as two-dimensional figures. He stated explicitly that the drawings of the zigzag wire and the rigid connector wire models were also meant to be two-dimensional figures. In a transitional segment, S2 drew a series of rods (figure 5.8) and thought about how they bend as weights are moved along them and as the length of the rod is taken to the limiting case (note that the bending is not drawn).

First, these drawings provide fixed representations of rods on which S2 performed imaginative experiments through imagining the weight, drawn in one location and annotated with an arrow, as it moves along a rod of various lengths (figure 5.8B) and is taken to the limit (figure 5.8D) and imagining the bend of the rod under these conditions. These experiments led again to the inference that the longer the rod, the greater the bend, reinforcing his earlier conclusion that the rod was not an adequate model for the spring, despite the fact that when a spring is stretched fully it is rodlike in appearance. That is, the bend of a rod does not exemplify the stretch of a spring. After this segment, S2 began discussing the geometry of a spring coil, which he said should be "irrelevant." He then had an insight that with rods, one "is always measuring in the vertical" and that maybe the way "the coiled spring unwinds makes for a difference in the frame of reference." This insight brought into play a constraint (T10) that a spring is coiled in the horizontal plane (has a horizontal component to its stretch) that had not previously played a role in his thinking.

He started thinking about a spring as a three-dimensional helix and then noted that an earlier diagram of an open coil (figure 5.9a) was meant to be of a helix, not a spiral.

He drew a spiral (figure 5.9b) and compared it with the geometry of an earlier diagram of stretched spring (figure 5.9c). In the initial context in which figure 5.9c was drawn, the spiral was meant to exemplify the uniform stretch of a spring. In this new reasoning context, it now exemplified the

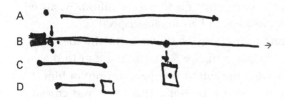

Figure 5.8
S2's drawings of a series of rods and weights.

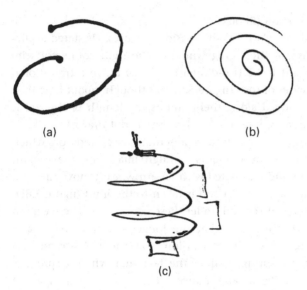

(a)   (b)

(c)

Figure 5.9
S2's explorations of three-dimensionality.

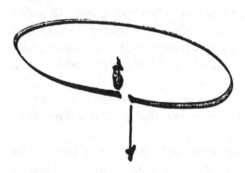

Figure 5.10
S2's drawing of a three-dimensional coil segment.

horizontal component of the curvature of a spring. Significantly, all subsequent figures were drawn in three-dimensional perspective.

S2's next diagram integrates the idea of stretch with the idea that it takes place in the horizontal plane (figure 5.10). In addition to drawing figure 5.10, he gestured drawing the coil in the space in front of him. The diagram of the open coil oriented in the horizontal plane was crucial to his insight about the torsion force operating in the stretch of a spring. Being represented in three-dimensional perspective affords a new kind of simulation—pushing or pulling down with vertical and horizontal components. S2 annotated the diagram with an arrow indicating the motion.

We have seen already from the mental animation and perceptual simulation literature that people are able to mentally simulate motions of the represented systems from a static diagram. In the course of using diagrams, people not only look at them, they often carry out physical actions on them, such as drawing on them, gesturing over them, and annotating them with arrows, just as S2 did. These physical actions can enhance the affordances of the diagram for mental simulation. Hegarty and Steinhoff (1997), for example, showed that people with low spatial ability, when allowed to draw and make notations on the diagram, were able to solve mental animation problems they were not able to otherwise. Notating a diagram with arrows not only provides orientation, but also can indicate causal relations and potential motion (Tversky et al. 2000). Arrows, then, can assist in simulation by aligning an external representation with the internal model of the reasoner. Further, diagrams can be augmented with language that indicates a simulation, as seen in both our exemplars.

S2 did not see the torsion effect straightaway, though. First he began to think about transmitting the stretch "from increment to increment of the spring" and bending a rod bit by bit into a spring coil, thus creating a hybrid rod–spring model. He drew a three-dimensional hexagonal spring coil—a representation that integrates features of rods and springs (figure 5.11, no. 11)—and this diagram led to an immediate perceptual inference that the rod segment "twists while stretching."

The segment expressing this insight in relation to the diagram is worth repeating in this context:

Just looking at this it occurs to me that when force is applied here [he draws a downward pointing arrow at the end of the line segment], you not only get a bend on this segment, but because there's a pivot here [points to the "X" in figure 5.11], you get a torsion effect—around here [points to the adjacent segment]. (121)
Aha!—Maybe the behavior of the spring has something to do with the twist forces [S2 moves his hands as if twisting an object, and continues to make either twisting or bending motions as the reasoning about the polygonal coil model unfolded]. That's a real interesting idea—that might be the key insight—that might be the key difference between this [points to flexible rod], which involves no torsion, and this [points to hexagonal coil]. (122)

The diagram of a hexagon colocates causal information about the relation between stretching and deformation, that is, it localizes the twist at the angular joint when one section is pulled down in the vertical plane, as marked by S2's drawing an "X" at the corner. It shows also that given the

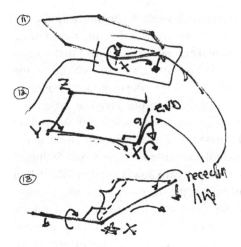

Figure 5.11
S2's drawing of three-dimensional hexagonal and square coil segments.

orientation of the figure in the horizontal plane, the twist would begin over again at each joint, which provides a different kind of stretching motion than with the earlier, two-dimensional rod–spring models. The diagrams of these models provide no indication of the mechanism that underlies the stretching behavior. The new diagram exemplifies the relational structure between the stretch of the coil and the twist of the rod segment, which literally affords seeing the twisting and facilitates the inference that the cause is a torsion force (presumably also now using some physics knowledge), and transforms the mental model he is reasoning with into one that includes a representation of torsion. S2 subsequently drew the square models to exaggerate the effect and extrapolated the inference to the spring coil as discussed in chapter 3, section 3.3.5.

5.2.3 Discovering Electromagnetic Wave Propagation
Historical documents seldom provide step-by-step accounts of reasoning processes as we have with problem-solving protocols; nevertheless, I have been arguing that the cognitive-historical method provides a means to make reasonable hypotheses in reconstructing such processes. Maxwell introduced the vortex–idle wheel diagram (Model 4, figure 5.2d) in conjunction with deriving the equations of electromagnetic induction. He directly coupled the derivations with the diagram. Maxwell's rendering of the vortex–idle wheel diagram in which the idle wheels are packed tightly around the vortices (thus the hexagonal shape) exemplifies a causal

relationship in which the motion of either idle wheels (representing electric current) or vortices (representing magnetism) causes motion in the other. That is, it exemplifies the causal structure of what he came to call a "connected system."

In the context of the electromagnetic analysis, the diagram might have been introduced to assist in conveying his complex dynamical model to potential readers, or to guide his own reasoning processes, or both. However, given the interval of months between the publication of that analysis and his analysis of electrostatic induction, we know for sure that Maxwell had the diagram at his disposal for the electrostatic analysis. Given the complexity of the mental model through which he was reasoning, it is reasonable to assume that the diagram helped in his reasoning, just as we saw with S2's simpler topological models. As such, we can look at the affordances of the diagram for his analysis of electrostatic induction and discovery of wave propagation in the electromagnetic aether.

On my interpretation of the historical records (section 2.2.3), reasoning about the potential motion at points of contact if elastic vortices and idle wheel particles were to be under stress from an external force (electrostatic) led directly to Maxwell's notion of "displacement current" and to the calculation of the velocity of its propagation through the medium (electromagnetic wave). Both the language of "displacement current" and the mathematical representation support this interpretation. It is the motion of the particles that represents a current, even if that motion is only a slight displacement. The causal structure of propagation of electrostatic forces in an aetherial medium is represented through topological changes when the vortices undergo elastic deformation as the idle wheels are urged forward by an applied force but remain in place. Propagation is a wave of distortion in the mechanical medium, produced as the displacement of electricity propagates through the elastic medium. Looking at the diagram (figure 5.2d) in light of Maxwell's interpretation, we can see this action as follows.

Maxwell specified a difference between conductors and dielectrics when he first introduced the idle wheel particles. In a conductor, they are free to move from vortex to vortex. In a dielectric, they can only rotate in place. The adjacency relation as represented in the diagram, coupled with the arrows drawn on it, exemplifies the idea that motion of either the idle wheel particles or the vortices causes motion in the other. One can infer from looking at the diagram that if the particles are not able to move out of place, then a force pressing them forward will create a distortion in the vortices (assuming they are elastic), which in turn will give rise to an oppositely oriented restoring force from the particles (action and reaction). The distortion will propagate through the medium until the system reaches equilibrium. This is the mechanism from which Maxwell derived the equations for electrostatic induction and the velocity of wave propagation.[14] Without the mechanism of the model, there is no basis on which to call the electrostatic displacement a "current," and without the model there is no basis for the minus sign in Maxwell's equation for representing displacement. The elastic restoring force should be oriented in the opposite direction to the electromotive force. The qualitative inferences about this complex set of causal relations are directly represented in the diagram, given Maxwell's modified interpretation of it for electrostatic phenomena, as are the mathematical derivations. It seems reasonable to assume it interacted with his mental model of the medium while he was reasoning about the phenomena, just as we saw with S2.

In the S2 and Maxwell exemplars, diagrams are representations of analogical models and participate in imaginative simulations of models. I want now to bring to the fore the "experimental" dimension of reasoning through simulating models.

5.3   Representation Simulation and Thought Experimenting

As I noted earlier, with creative model-based reasoning it is often artificial to treat analogy, imagery, and simulation as separate processes, since each is implicated in the other. In the exemplars, for instance, predictions are made on the basis of simulative enactments of the behaviors of models, constructed using analogy and facilitated by imagistic representations. On my account, these kinds of simulations lie on a continuum between mundane simulations, such as of how to get a chair through a doorway, and carefully crafted thought experiments by scientists (such as Einstein's thought experiments about the experiences of an observer in a chest in outer space or falling to earth in an elevator). Clement, too, argues that S2's simulations of motion of the models should be considered thought experiments in that they are acts "of predicting the behavior of an untested, concrete, but absent system" (Clement 2003, 4). On simulating the stretching of the imaginary hexagonal rod–spring model, S2 predicted that the segments would twist as the hexagonal spring stretched, and, through further inferences, came to predict that torsion is what keeps the stretch of a spring uniformly distributed.

In some instances, such as Maxwell's model, the system is not only absent, but physically implausible as a whole. Yet, significant predictions are made on the basis of the model that contribute to solving the real-world problem. For instance, on simulating the motion of the vortices packed together in the medium, Maxwell predicted that friction among them would cause jamming. This led to the realization that the initial model was an inadequate representation of continuous motion in a mechanical medium. Note that the "experimental outcome," as we saw, did not in itself provide the solution to the problem. However, it presented a problem that, when solved by introducing the idle wheel particles through further reasoning, provided a means of representing the dynamical relations between currents and magnetism. So, too, full-blown thought experiments often only point out the problem. Even more significantly, simulating the behavior of the vortex–idle wheel model undergoing deformation, he predicted the velocity of propagation of a wave of distortion in the medium would be the same as of light. This led to the prediction that electromagnetic waves propagate at the speed of light (thus, if correct, that field processes exist in the space surrounding bodies), to the hypothesis that light is an electromagnetic phenomenon, and to the search, experimentally, for the predicted electromagnetic waves.

Some time ago I introduced the idea that thought experimenting was a species of *simulative model-based reasoning*, the cognitive basis of which is the capacity for mental modeling (Nersessian 1991, 1992 a,b).[15] My hypothesis, then as now, is that executing a thought experiment involves constructing and simulating a mental model to determine what would happen if specified manipulations were to take place. It is a species of reasoning rooted in the ability to imagine, anticipate, visualize, and reexperience from memory. It might be possible to reconstruct a thought experiment as an argument in propositional form, as John Norton has demonstrated for many cases (Norton 1991, 2004), but such propositional articulation at most codifies a reasoning process that already has been carried out by other means. That is, the mental model needs to have been constructed and simulated in order for the propositions that make up the argument to be identified. Thought-experimental narratives, when devised after the initial experimenting, are designed to evoke reasoning processes that parallel the original mental execution of the experiment. Contemporary real-world experimental narratives are much less story-like, but they, too, are not presented in logical form.[16] Real-world and thought-experimental narratives aim at enabling the expected audience to reason through either carrying out an experiment or executing it imaginatively.

The difference, of course, between real and imagined experiments is that humans have a seemingly boundless capacity for fictive imagining. What distinguishes young Einstein's imaginings of traveling beside a light wave from young Nancy's imaginings of riding a pink elephant in a fairyland world? What gives epistemic import to the former but not the latter? I think there is no definitive answer that will distinguish all cases, but the basic response is that why an experiment carried out in thought has potential import for science is rooted in the problem-solving context in which it is conducted and the nature of the goals the reasoner wants to achieve. Einstein, even at that tender age, was addressing what he thought to be a problem in Maxwell's electromagnetic theory, and he wanted to understand perplexing features of his understanding of the implications of that representation. Nancy was bored with her classes and simply daydreaming. Customarily, the scientific thought experiment is designed to examine aspects of a way of representing real-world phenomena for the purposes of determining what consequences follow from that way of representing them. Just as with real-world experiments, scientific thought experiments are selective constructions and make clear which aspects of the world can be discounted. In Einstein's experiment of an observer in a room being pulled upward in outer space, the audience implicitly understands to disregard such real-world considerations as that the person would die from lack of oxygen, the nature of the "being" existing in outer space that is pulling a rope attached to the chest, and so forth. What we are directed to focus on is that the observer's experience of the behavior of objects (including himself) would be the same as if he were stationary on Earth. This leads to the inference that the laws of physics are the same in uniformly accelerated frames of reference and in homogeneous gravitational fields (generalized principle of relativity).

S2 conveyed his model simulations through drawings, language, and gestures. Maxwell instructed his audience to imagine his drawings of models as animated in specific ways. The predominant data for analyzing the nature of thought experiments, however, are in the form of well-crafted narratives used to convey how to conduct them after the experimenters have determined that the experiments achieve the desired outcomes. I take the ubiquity of the narrative form of presentation to indicate that something about the connection of this kind of reasoning with narration is cognitively important.

5.3.1 Thought-experimental Narratives

We saw in chapter 4, section 4.4.1, that there is an extensive literature on comprehending and reasoning with narratives that supports the interpretation that people construct mental models of the situations depicted by the narratives and make inferences through manipulating these, rather than by performing logical operations on proposition-like representations. That is, the referent of the text of the narrative is an internal model of the situation rather than an internal description. Even though scientific thought experiments are more complex than the cases of reasoning investigated in the mental modeling literature, it seems reasonable to assume that these narratives would serve much the same functions. My hypothesis is that the carefully crafted thought-experimental narrative leads to the construction of a mental model of a kind of situation, and that simulating consequences of the situation affords epistemic access to specific aspects of a way or ways of representing the world. I construe "narrative" sufficiently broadly to encompass the range from straightforward descriptions, such as Galileo's sparse description of imagining two stones of different weights, joined together and falling (in exploring the possible differences in the rates of falling bodies), to more elaborate "stories" such as his description of an artist drawing on a ship while on a voyage from Venice to Alexandretta (in exploring whether one can perceive common motion). The thought-experimental narrative describes a sequence of events that calls upon the audience to imagine a dynamic scene, one that unfolds in time. The function of the narrative is to guide the reader to construct a model of the situation described by it and to make inferences through simulating the events and processes depicted by the model.

Thought-experimental models afford a means of investigating the consequences—conceptual or empirical—that follow from a way of representing the world. In themselves they usually do not present the solution, but often they indicate avenues of possible change. Here again the notion of exemplification is useful in thinking about the cognitive function of thought-experimental narratives. Elgin (1996; in press) argues that fictional narratives afford insight, for instance about human relations, when the stories are crafted so as to exemplify the requisite aspects of human relations, such as the dynamics of family life within the claustrophobic atmosphere of a nineteenth-century English village. To this I would add that the fictional narrative aids in constructing a mental model that refers to and instantiates these relational structures. Thought-experimental narratives, too, are crafted so as to focus attention on features relevant to epistemic goals of the problem-solving context. A good experiment also makes clear which features instantiated in the model are germane and which can be discounted. Norton (1991) notes that often "irrelevant particulars" are instantiated in the model—for instance that the physicist is drunk or drugged when he is first put into the chest. Rather than being irrelevant, however, in many instances they serve to focus attention on crucial features of the experiment; in this case, that the physicist has no way of knowing where he is—on Earth or in space.

By exemplifying dynamical situations of a certain kind and following out their consequences, the simulation model affords experimental access to previously unnoticed consequences of representations. The cognitive capacity for generic abstraction enables understanding the specific experimental situation—mental or physical—as representing situations of *this kind*—as belonging to this class of phenomena. The narrative provides a means through which to grasp insights and gain understanding about representing phenomena in this way, and warrants pursuing the consequences to which the experimental outcomes lead, as with a real-world experiment.

Some instances of actual thought experiments can serve to illustrate how exemplification works in thought experimental narratives. Galileo's thought experiment of relative motion on a moving ship is developed over several pages, so I present only snippets. He proposes imagining (Galilei 1632, 171–172):

Sargredo: There just occurred to me a certain fantasy which passed through my imagination one day while I was sailing to Aleppo, where I was going as consul for our country. Perhaps it may be of some help in explaining how this motion in common is nonoperative and remains as if nonexistent to everything that participates in it.

Simplicius: The novelty of the things I am hearing makes me not merely tolerant but curious; please go on.

Sarg.: If the point of a pen had been on the ship during my whole voyage from Venice to Alexandretta and had had the property of leaving visible marks of its whole trip, what trace—what mark—what line would it have left?

Simp.: It would have left a line extending from Venice to there; not perfectly straight—or rather, not lying in the perfect arc of a circle—but more or less fluctuating according as the vessel would now and again have rocked. . . .

Sarg.: So if that fluctuation of the waves were taken away and the motion of the vessel were calm and tranquil, the true and precise motion of the pen point would have been an arc of a perfect circle. Now if I had had that same pen continually in my hand and had moved it only a little sometimes this way or that, what alteration should I have brought to the main extent of the line?

Simp.: Less than that which would be given to a straight line a thousand yards long which deviated from absolute straightness here and there by a flea's eye.

Sarg: Then if an artist had begun drawing with that pen on a sheet of paper when we left the port and had continued doing so all the way to Alexandretta, he would have been able to draw from the pen's motion a whole narrative of many figures . . . the artist's own actions . . . would have been conducted exactly the same as if the ship had been standing still.

The context of this experiment is Galileo's discussion of the Copernican hypothesis that the Earth is in motion around the sun. From it we are supposed to infer that we cannot observe directly motion that objects attached to the Earth share with the Earth. Understanding what claims can be made about the behavior of all objects that share a motion on the basis of a simulation of specific objects derives from understanding how the exemplified features of the one situation transfer across all such situations, not through inductive generalization. The ship's motion exemplifies the motion of the Earth along a curve over a significant distance; that is, in the thought-experimental model, the imaginary ship's motion is to have the same relation with respect to the imagined Earth as the motion of the Earth has with respect to space. Call it "motion$_1$."

The exact particulars of the depiction of the narrative are not significant, such as being on a ship and of traveling from Venice to Alexandretta, but serve to provoke the audience's imagination. The narrative is crafted in such a way that one understands that these are not in themselves significant, but can serve to focus attention on the quite relevant feature(s); here it is motion$_1$. The pen exemplifies the motion of any body moving along with the Earth, and thus sharing in motion$_1$. In the first instance, were we able to trace the motion of the pen (body) through the water (heavens) we would see a curved line (discounting possible fluctuations due to waves in the water as irrelevant—the Earth does not encounter waves). The same would hold if someone riding on the ship (observer on moving Earth) were to just hold onto the pen, so the person shares in the motion$_1$ of the pen. However, from the perspective of the artist on the ship holding the pen and drawing (making local motion$_2$), it traces only lines with respect to its motion$_2$ as evidenced on the paper. In conclusion there is only evidence of motion$_2$; no evidence of the shared motion$_1$ can be detected. The larger conclusion Galileo wants the audience to infer is that there is no inconsistency in maintaining that the Earth is in motion and yet observers on the Earth do not experience that motion.

Einstein presented his thought experiment of the behavior of bodies in a chest in space in several forms (including falling elevator versions); an early version from 1916 is as follows (Einstein 1961, 66–67):

We imagine a large portion of empty space, so far removed from stars and other appreciable masses, that we have before us approximately the conditions required by the fundamental law of Galilei. It is then possible to choose a Galilean reference-body for this part of space (world) relative to which points at rest remain at rest and points in motion continue permanently in uniform rectilinear motion. As reference-body let us imagine a spacious chest resembling a room with an observer inside who is equipped with apparatus. Gravitation naturally does not exist for this observer. He must fasten himself with strings to the floor, otherwise the slightest impact against the floor will cause him to rise slowly towards the ceiling of the room.

To the middle of the lid of the chest is fixed externally a hook with a rope attached and now a "being" (what kind of a being is immaterial to us) begins pulling at this with a constant force. The chest together with the observer then begin to move "upwards" with a uniformly accelerated motion. . . . But how does the man in the chest regard the process? The acceleration of the chest will be transmitted to him by reaction of the floor of the chest. . . . He is then standing in the chest in exactly the same way as anyone stands in a room of a house on our earth. If he releases a body which he previously had in his hand, the acceleration of the chest will no longer be transmitted to this body, and for this reason the body will fall to the floor of the chest with an accelerated relative motion. . . .

Relying on his knowledge of the gravitational field, the man in the chest will thus come to the conclusion that he and the chest are in a gravitational field that is constant with regard to time. Of course he will be puzzled for a moment as to why the chest does not fall in this gravitational field. Just then, however, he discovers the hook in the middle of the chest and the rope attached to it, and consequently he comes to the conclusion that the chest is suspended at rest in the gravitational field.

Ought we to smile at the man and say that he errs in his conclusion? I do not believe we ought to if we wish to remain consistent; we must rather admit that his mode of grasping the situation violates neither reason nor known mechanical laws. . . . as a result we have gained a powerful argument for a generalized postulate of relativity.

The context of this experiment is Einstein's discussion of whether the principle of equivalence need be restricted to only inertial systems (Galilean invariance). In the initial situation, the chest exemplifies any inertial system with all its consequent features; that is, the thought-experimental model of the chest represents a container in which objects move in a straight line unless impeded by a force, such as that of the strings on the observer's ankles. In the second situation, the uniformly accelerating chest exemplifies any frame of reference in which objects undergo accelerated relative motion. The action of the "being" pulling the rope exemplifies one means of uniformly accelerated motion. The chest could have been made to accelerate by any means. The experiences of the observer in the chest are to him the same as if he were in a homogeneous gravitational field, and so he infers, on seeing the hook, that he is suspended at rest in one. This inference highlights another feature of the "spacious chest resembling a room" that might not have been noticed at first: the observer cannot see outside of it to determine where he is and what bodies might be in his vicinity. As those who criticized Einstein's conclusion as not pertaining to the real world pointed out, gravitational fields in nature are distinguished from accelerated frames in that the fields have sources. So, the experiment depends crucially on the representation of the observer as not being able to see any objects around him, and thus, some argued, is not in itself sufficient to conclude the equivalence.

The outcomes of thought experiments are in need of interpretation. As with these examples, often the insights thought experiments lead to are in the form of problems such as that the representations lead to contradictory or physically impossible situations. This warrants thinking that something is wrong with a certain way of representing the world and investigating the problem indicated by the outcome. The significance of a thought experiment, however, can be a matter of prolonged debate within the community. Galileo's thought experiment does not lead directly to the Copernican hypothesis. The implications of Einstein's thought experiment were debated for a considerable period. Thought-experimenting takes place within a problem-solving context, and needs to conform to the constraints of that context. How acceptable an outcome is depends on the understandings that frame it. As with real experiments, the outcome does not stand on its own, but requires interpretation and further investigation—empirical or conceptual.

On a mental modeling account, then, a thought-experimental model is a conceptual system representing the physical system that is being reasoned about. More than one instantiation or realization of a situation described in the narrative is possible. The constructed model need only be of *the same kind* with respect to salient dimensions of target phenomena. Thought-experimental models embody and comply with the represented constraints of the phenomena being reasoned about. Constraints used in constructing and manipulating models are conditioned by experience and by current theoretical understanding. Operations on thought-experimental models require that transformations be consistent with the constraints of the domain, which can be tacit or explicit for the experimenter. What transformations are possible and legitimate derive from the constraints. Causal coherence, spatial structure, and mathematical consistency are examples of kinds of constraints. Inferences are derived directly through manipulations of the model. The models represent demonstratively (as opposed to descriptively). Whether it is a good model is evaluated according to how well the situation conforms to the kind of phenomena it is supposed to represent and the usefulness of the inferences that flow from simulating it.

In his influential 1964 essay, Thomas Kuhn characterized thought-experimenting as "one of the essential analytical tools which are deployed during crises and which then help to promote basic conceptual reform" (Kuhn 1977, 263). The historical record does indeed show the preponderance of thought experiments in periods of conceptual change in science. But, to understand why it is an "essential analytical tool" requires a fundamental revision of how we conceive of conceptual change—one that differs from both traditional and Kuhnian accounts. Chapter 6 addresses how this and other forms of model-based reasoning are productive means of conceptual innovation.

5.4 Model-based Reasoning

Having considered the practices of analogical, imagistic, and simulative modeling to some extent separately, I will now extract several key common ingredients that will be taken into the final chapter on conceptual change. The problem-solving processes we have considered in which these practices are employed involve constructing, manipulating, evaluating, and adapting models that are built to selectively represent target phenomena. Models are constructed to satisfy constraints drawn from the target domain, from one or more source domains, and that can arise from the model itself. These constraints can be provided by means of linguistic, formulaic, and imagistic informational formats, including equations, texts, diagrams, pictures, maps, physical models, and kinesthetic and auditory experiences. Enhanced understanding of the target problem that has been obtained through the modeling process can lead to recognizing as salient target constraints previously unnoticed or disregarded. Simulation can be used to examine how constraints interact, to produce new constraints, and to enable evaluation of behaviors, constraint satisfaction, and other factors.

Model-based reasoning utilizes various forms of abstraction, such as limiting case, idealization, generalization, and generic abstraction. Abstraction via generic modeling ("generic abstraction") plays a highly significant role in the generation and integration of constraints, and in delimiting the scope of inferences. Model-based reasoning makes use of both highly specific domain knowledge and knowledge of abstract general principles, as well as knowledge of how to make appropriate abstractions.

Evaluation and revision are crucial components of model-based reasoning. These processes make use of structural, behavioral, and/or functional constraint satisfaction. In particular, a highly salient criterion is that the model be of the *same kind* with respect to salient dimensions of target phenomena. I have used the notion that the models exemplify the requisite relational structures and processes as a way of interpreting how "same kind" is the feature that warrants transferring insight and understanding derived from thinking with the models to the real-world phenomena.

6 Creativity in Conceptual Change

Language can become a screen that stands between the thinker and reality. That is the reason why true creativity often starts where language ends.
—Arthur Koestler, *The Act of Creation*[1]

[A] concept is not an isolated, ossified changeless formation, but an active part of the intellectual process, constantly engaged in serving communication, understanding, and problem solving.
—Lev Vygotsky, *Language and Thought*

How are vague, preliminary notions about how to understand phenomena transformed into scientific concepts? The proposal of this book is that in many instances novel concepts are constructed using model-based reasoning. The view provided of conceptual innovation, then, is that it stems from extended, often incremental, modeling processes—even if there might be "aha!" moments along the way.

No doubt methods of conceptual innovation comprise more than the kinds of reasoning we have been considering. Nevertheless, progress on understanding a key, largely neglected, component of conceptual change can be made through examining how model-based reasoning serves to create novel candidate representations. Although conceptual change in science is a phenomenon that takes place across communities, it is primarily individual scientists who create the conceptual innovations that are investigated, further articulated, and adopted by communities. Thus an accounting is needed of the details of individual reasoning in problem solving—where problem solving in science must always be understood as situated within social and cultural contexts that provide conceptual and material resources for, and constraints on, it—and of the cognitive structures enabling such reasoning.

6.1 Model-based Reasoning: The Argument Thus Far

The major conclusion of the argument is that *model-based reasoning is genuine reasoning*. It is not an ancillary aid to reasoning carried out by logical manipulations of propositional representations. Inferences are made through constructing and manipulating models that are structural, behavioral, or functional analog models of target phenomena. Models are constructed to satisfy constraints deriving from the target and source domains, and those that might emerge from the model itself. Constraints comprise, among others, the spatial, temporal, causal, functional, categorical, and mathematical. Constraint satisfaction limits the number of possible ways of proceeding, without rigidly specifying the moves one can make within the space of possibilities. Constructed models are dynamic in that they afford making inferences through simulation processes.

Model-based reasoning is ampliative and can be creative. Through it understanding is enlarged or deepened, often in ways that lead to novel insights and even conceptual change. When creative, it lies on a continuum with usage in ordinary problem solving. It makes use of cognitive processes underlying ordinary model-based inference, including mental modeling and analogical, imagistic, and simulative processes. When used in science, likewise, it lies on a continuum with ordinary usage. Differences in usage arise largely from the nature of the problem and the problem situation. Highly creative uses, such as S2's, can arise in the context of problems that cannot be solved by direct mapping from any analogical source known—or that is recalled—by the reasoner. Scientific uses, such as Maxwell's, are likely to be more explicit and reflective than ordinary uses because the problem situation comprises deep knowledge of a repertoire of methods, domain-specific knowledge, and significant problem-solving experience.[2]

Model-based reasoning involves bootstrapping, which consists of cycles of construction, simulation, evaluation, and adaptation of models that serve as interim interpretations of the target problem. I outline the bootstrapping processes here and elaborate these in section 6.2 on conceptual innovation. They are as follows. *Model construction* starts with a rudimentary understanding of the target phenomena, sufficient enough to furnish initial constraints. These constraints, together with the goals of the problem solving, guide the selection of an analogical source domain and the selection of relevant constraints within it. Selection of a source domain can involve imagistic and simulative processes. An initial model is created through which the problem solver attempts to combine and integrate constraints from both domains. Selecting and merging constraints makes use of processes of *abstraction*, such as idealization, approximation, limiting case, and generic modeling. *Simulation* produces new states through manipulating the model. It enables examining the interaction of constraints in the model, inferring outcomes, and making predictions. These processes can make salient constraints of target, source, or model not previously noticed or regarded as salient. *Evaluation* involves making a comparison between selected features of the model and the target as determined by the problem. Initial evaluation criteria center around determining if the model represents all salient constraints of the target (is of the *same kind*), which requires establishing an initial mapping between target and model. If it does, then the problem solution in the model can be transferred to the target, where it is evaluated according to the problem requirements—for instance, it provides a satisfactory explanatory mechanism; it enables a satisfactory mathematical representation; it yields testable empirical hypotheses; and so forth. If a model were fully satisfactory in providing a problem solution, the process could stop here. However, models are frequently modified or extended in problem-solving processes, furnishing a series of building blocks leading toward a problem solution. *Adaptation* takes place according to the enhanced understanding of target, source, and model constraints. This might involve selecting an additional source domain.

Throughout the bootstrapping processes, *model-based reasoning involves selectivity*. Selectivity enables bracketing (potentially) irrelevant features and focuses attention on those relevant to the problem-solving context. Relevant constraints need to be determined for target and source domains. Abstractive and evaluative processes disregard irrelevant factors. Constructed models can instantiate irrelevant factors, as we discussed with thought experiments, but to reason correctly via a model requires recognizing these as scaffolding for the cognitively germane factors. I have argued that the germane factors are those that are exemplified in the model.

Clearly, *model-based reasoning is closely bound up with analogy*. Models are built and evaluated on the basis of relational comparisons. Productive mappings and transfer between models and target need to meet criteria established by cognitive scientists for analogy. However, on my account, the bootstrapping processes of model-based reasoning go beyond what can be accommodated by existing theories of analogy. Understanding model-based reasoning demands an accounting of the processes of representation-building, and of the roles of imagistic and simulative processes in reasoning.

6.2 Conceptual Innovation

Section 6.1 provides an account of model-based reasoning that covers its usage generally. I now return to the central problem of creativity in conceptual change, rephrased in light of the analysis thus far: *What features of model-based reasoning make it a particularly effective means of conceptual innovation?* My account of conceptual change is not intended as only of a kind of individual cognitive change, but also of a kind of representational change within the scientific community, as is customarily associated with "revolutionary" changes in theory (such as of "mass" in Newtonian mechanics to "mass" in the special theory of relativity). These are public representations shared by members of a community. Talking of concepts provides a means of bridging the psychological and the community phenomena. Concepts are a basic way through which humans represent the world. They categorize experiences and take note of relationships, differences, and interconnections among them. For the individual, concepts figure in a range of cognitive phenomena including memory, inference, problem solving, language comprehension, and belief systems, to name a few.[3] Scientific concepts provide systematic representations through which individuals and communities understand, explain, and make predictions about phenomena.

The exemplars developed in chapters 2 and 3 furnish substance to the account of bootstrapping just outlined, as it applies to conceptual innovation. Maxwell's model-based reasoning provided ways of representing kinetic energy and potential energy—necessary components of a concept of field—that neither he nor physics possessed when he began. He bootstrapped to a field representation starting from a quite general notion that electric and magnetic processes take place in the region surrounding bodies and from a few specific constraints deriving from experimental research on and theorizing about electricity and magnetism in his problem situation. S2's model-based reasoning provided a way of representing the mechanism underlying the uniform stretch of a spring, which he did not possess when he began. He evidently had a notion of torsion, but not associated with springs. He bootstrapped to the physics representation of "spring" as including "torsion," starting from an intuitive notion of spring and a few specific constraints deriving from the problem. Each went through several iterations of constructing models by drawing on representational resources in analogical source domains outside of the target domain.[4] These imaginary hybrid models merge constraints arising from the target, the source, and the model.

I outline my account of how such bootstrapping leads to conceptual innovation as follows, and elaborate in the remainder of this chapter. As a form of representation, a concept specifies sets of constraints which can be used to generate members of a class of models. Concept formation and change is a process of generating new, or modifying existing, constraints (this covers both of what are customarily referred to as "weak" and "strong"—or "revolutionary"—conceptual change). Model-based reasoning is prevalent in conceptual innovation in science because it is a highly effective means of making evident, and focusing attention on, constraints of existing representational systems, of selectively abstracting constraints and bypassing others, and of facilitating their integration from multiple domains. The constructed models provide scaffolding for bootstrapping toward a satisfactory representation. Through these processes truly novel combinations of constraints that correspond to heretofore unrepresented structures and behaviors can emerge—those which, in H-creative cases, cannot be represented within existing conceptual structures.

6.2.1 Concepts

In previous work I addressed the issue of the format of the representation of a concept. I argued against the classical "necessary and sufficient conditions" view and in favor of more flexible notions consistent with empirical evidence on human categorization, generally, under development in cognitive research, such as "schemata," "dynamic frames," and "idealized cognitive models."[5] There is as yet no consensus concept of "concept" in cognitive science or in philosophy of science. Formal proposals and critiques of alternative views are usually dependent on the purposes concepts serve in a particular analysis. From the perspective of scientific change, the classical view of representation is inadequate in that it allows at most for change through replacement, not for change through modifications of the sort I call "descendants," such as the concept of "inertia" from Galileo to Newton or "field" from Faraday to Einstein. To complicate things further, features of concepts that appear to have been eliminated, such as "aether," can be cast as having been *absorbed* by other concepts, in this case "field" and "space-time," in whose formation the historical evidence indicates they played a role. For the present analysis, the format issue can be bypassed by stipulating only that whatever the format of a concept, concepts specify constraints for generating members of a class of models.

The "dynamic frames" notion of Lawrence Barsalou (1999) helps to illustrate the idea that concepts specify constraints. One advantage of thinking of concepts in this way is that Barsalou has shown how his theory

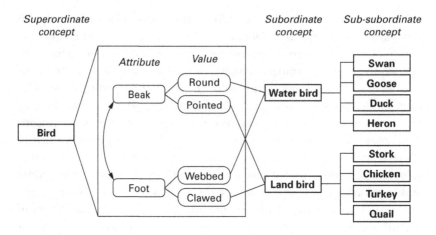

Superordinate concept *Subordinate concept* *Sub-subordinate concept*

Figure 6.1
Partial dynamic frame of Ray's concept of bird (1678). Arrows indicate constraints. Reproduced from Andersen, Barker, and Chen (2006), figure 21, p. 73, reprinted with permission of Cambridge University Press.

of perceptual symbol systems, which we discussed in conjunction with mental modeling, supports this earlier notion of categorization. A second advantage is that Hanne Andersen, Peter Barker, and Xiang Chen have made excellent use of this notion in further articulating Thomas Kuhn's ideas about concepts, incommensurability, and conceptual change. The results of their research are summarized and elaborated in a recent book, *The Cognitive Structure of Scientific Revolutions* (Andersen, Barker, and Chen 2006). Although not all scientific concepts readily yield to a dynamic frame analysis (see Nersessian and Andersen 1997, 2000), I will use a case they developed to illustrate the notion that concepts specify constraints and conceptual innovation involves changing and creating new constraints.

Figure 6.1 provides a partial representation of an early concept of bird as formulated in the first ornithological taxonomy by J. Ray in 1678. Birds were classified, simply, as either water birds or land birds. As the frame shows, the attributes beak and foot are mutually constraining. That means, for instance, that a round beak requires a webbed foot and a pointed beak requires a clawed foot. The discovery of screamers created a problem. Screamers have pointed beaks and webbed feet.[6] Thus, they violate the constraint specified by the concept of bird as then understood.

A popular taxonomy developed by G. Sundevall in the 1830s accommodated this and other anomalies now classified as "grallatores" through

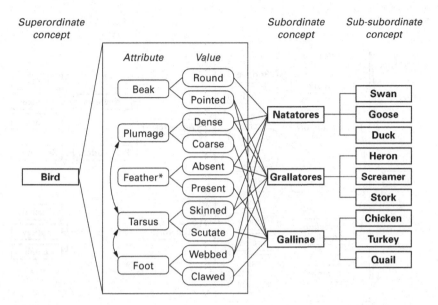

Figure 6.2
Partial dynamic frame of Sundevall's concept of bird (1835). Arrows indicate constraints. Reproduced from Andersen, Barker, and Chen (2006), figure 22, p. 74, reprinted with permission of Cambridge University Press. The attribute feather refers to the existence of the fifth secondary.

increasing the number of relevant attributes, which altered and added constraints to the concept of bird (figure 6.2). Andersen, Barker, and Chen (2006) argue that this is a weak form of conceptual change since the new representation is an elaboration that, while making possible new property combinations, is consistent with the significant features of the old classifications. In particular, it captures the previous dissimilarity relations among water birds and land birds. However, post-Darwinian taxonomies required revolutionary conceptual change. They argue that the popular taxonomy of H. Gadow not only introduces a different set of attributes but that the constraint relations among attributes reflect the new Darwinian assumption that similarities in anatomical features show a common origin (figure 6.3). Thus there is incommensurability between the pre- and post-Darwinian concepts of bird. I refer the reader to their book for an elaboration of the argument.

Thinking about concepts in this limited fashion affords insights into how model-based reasoning is a productive strategy in bringing about such change. On my account, conceptual innovation involves processes of

Superordinate   Subordinate
   concept   concept

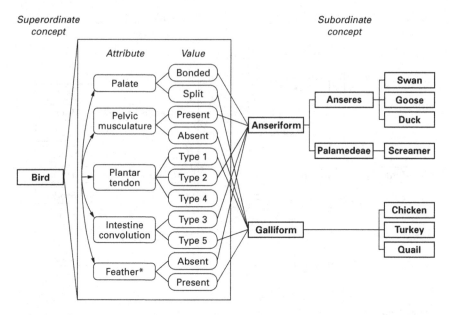

Figure 6.3
Partial dynamic frame of Gadow's concept of bird (1893). Arrows indicate constraints. Reproduced from Andersen, Barker, and Chen (2006), figure 35, p. 88, reprinted with permission of Cambridge University Press.

modifying existing sets of constraints or generating entirely novel sets of constraints. Models are constructed, evaluated, and adapted to satisfy constraints. The objective in model construction is to arrive at a model of the same kind with respect to the salient constraints of the target problem. Analogical, visual, and simulative processes are effective means of abstracting and integrating constraints from multiple domains. Through their interaction novel combinations (H-creative or P-creative) can emerge.

As we saw in the exemplars, the known constraints of the domain under investigation are not sufficient to enable the problem solution, and so analogical sources are drawn upon. But here, too, no direct problem solution can be found. That is, neither domain alone contains the representational resources sufficient to solve the problem. Rather, the analogical source domains serve as sources of constraints for constructing novel, hybrid models—in these instances, models that are simultaneously electromagnetic and continuum mechanical representations or rod and spring representations. The model representations are specific, but the inferences made from them about the target phenomena require thinking of the representation at a level of generality sufficient to capture the constraints of a whole class of phenomena. Processes of abstraction, then, are key to the selective use and discovery of constraints, as are changes in representation afforded by analogy-making, visualization, and thought-experimenting. I consider in turn selectivity through processes of abstraction and selectivity through representational change.

6.2.2 Abstraction

That there are different kinds of abstractive processes is not often addressed in philosophy of science or cognitive science. As we saw in chapters 2 and 3, various kinds of abstractive processes play a role in model construction, in particular: idealization, approximation, limiting case, and generic abstraction. These provide different means of selectively focusing on features relevant to the particular case of problem solving while suppressing information that could inhibit the process. Suppression and selective highlighting of features provide ways of representing the problem in a cognitively tractable manner. Most important for conceptual innovation, they enable integration of information from different sources.

Idealization is a common strategy for relating mathematical representations to phenomena. Thinking of the sides of a triangle as having zero width, from the perspective of a geometrical figure, or the mass of a body as concentrated at a point, from the perspective of determining motion, allows strict application of mathematical formulae. Once mathematized, the idealization provides a point of departure from which to add information about real-world phenomena as deemed relevant to a problem. Limiting-case abstractions involve extrapolation or reduction to a minimum. This can include creating an idealized representation that extrapolates a value to zero, but it also includes reductions of the sort that Maxwell made in considering the behavior of one vortex, or that S2 made in reducing a spring to one coil. With respect to the problems at hand, each deemed that one segment of a repeating object had all the requisite features relevant to the problem at that stage of the analysis. However, in comparing the rod to a spring, initially, it was important that the representation of the spring include multiple coils in order for S2 to represent the difference in the way these stretch. Maxwell was able to make considerable progress in giving mathematical expression to various magnetic phenomena by selectively attending to only one vortex. To address the relations between electricity and magnetism, though, he needed to take into account the relations among vortices in the medium, which brought to the fore friction as a problem with the model as a mechanical system.

Approximation provides a means of discounting the relevance of differences. A standard approximation in physics is the "first-order approximation" used when applying a mathematical representation. Basically it makes the assumption that any higher-order effects are likely to be irrelevant or to be so complex as to make the analysis intractable. For instance, a laminar flow—one without currents or eddies—provides a first-order approximation sufficient for solving problems pertaining to many fluid dynamical phenomena. When he derived the mathematical relations between the vortices and the idle wheels, Maxwell assumed the vortices to approximate rigid pseudospheres on rotation (see figure 2.15). The approximation assumed that any actual deviation would be negligible for capturing the mathematical relations among them and the idle wheels. The idealization that they are rigid aided in that process, but addressing electrostatic phenomena required him to add the information that in such a medium they would need to be elastic. This was necessary for representing the reaction of the medium to an impressed force. Including elasticity in the constraints eventually yielded the insight that wave propagation in the medium approximates that of light. S2's understanding that a polygon approximates a circle in the limit where the side segments become infinitely small enabled him to discount any differences in the relation between twisting and stretching of a hexagonal, square, or circular coil. The polygonal representations exaggerate the twisting mechanism, which allowed him, literally, to see the twist in the hexagonal coil and understand that the inference transfers to the spring since, in the limit of no sides (smooth curve), torsion would distribute evenly.

Although different kinds of abstraction often occur in tandem, differentiating them serves to call attention to a kind of abstraction that is especially productive in merging constraints from multiple sources, and thus is highly significant for the problem of conceptual innovation. For instance, in considering the behavior of a physical system, such as a spring, scientists often draw a specific instance, but then reason with it as without specificity as to the number and width of coils. To reason about it as a generic simple harmonic oscillator requires, further, suppressing features of its spring-like structure and behaviors. I have called this "abstraction via generic modeling," or, simply, generic abstraction.[7] In model-based reasoning, constraints drawn from different sources need to be understood at a level of generality sufficient for retrieval, integration, and transfer. Further, generic abstraction gives generality to inferences made from the specific models that are constructed. As Berkeley noted, one cannot imagine a *triangle-in-general* but only some specific instance. However, in considering what it has in

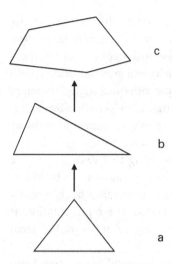

Figure 6.4
Abstraction via generic modeling.

common with all triangles, we are able to view the specific triangle as lacking specificity in the lengths of the sides and degrees of the angles.

The notion of generic abstraction is easily illustrated with an example, following Polya (1954). The reader should look at figure 6.4 as I construct the example. In Euclidean geometry the idealized triangle is understood as having lines that meet at a point, enclose a space, but have no width. The representation of a Euclidean triangle can be understood as of a specific kind, such as isosceles (figure 6.4a), for which the equivalence of two sides and of the angles opposite them needs to be specified. That representation, or any other representation of a triangle (e.g., figure 6.4b), can be understood to represent a triangle-in-general (or "generic" triangle), for which it needs only to be specified that the sides enclosing the angles are three in number. To make inferences about the generic triangle requires selectively suppressing information in the specific representation. To understand a representation as that of a generic polygon (figure 6.4c), the number of sides and angles needs to be understood as unspecified, even though a specific number are represented. Generic abstraction, then, consists of selectively suppressing information instantiated in a representation, so as to make inferences that pertain only to the generic case.

What I am trying to capture with the notion of making inferences through generic abstraction is similar to what mathematicians call making inferences through "generalization," but since this designation runs the risk of being conflated with "generalization" in logic, which is yet another form of reasoning, I have used "generic abstraction." To generalize in logic is to focus on specific features of one or a few instances and apply these to all instances. Using the above illustration, a logical generalization would be the inference "this isosceles triangle has equal opposite angles; therefore all isosceles triangles have equal opposite angles." A generic abstraction would suppress specific features of an instance of a triangle and yield an inference such as "the degrees of angles of the Euclidean triangle admit of many combinations, constrained only by summing to 180 degrees." The relation between a generic model and the specific instantiation is akin to the distinction between a type and an instance. Generality in representation is achieved by interpreting the components of the representation as standing for object, property, relation, or behavior types rather than instances of these.

Several instances of generic abstraction were discussed in chapters 2 and 3. In both exemplars, the nature of the problem and the reasoning context required that inferences made from the models be understood as applying to members of classes of phenomena. S2 constructed specific representations of polygonal coils—a hexagon and a square—but understood the inference that these would twist when stretched to hold for polygonal coils with any number of sides. The limiting case would be no sides, or a circular coil. Thus S2 immediately understood that the inference about torsion would apply to circular coils. This inference resulted in the change in his concept of spring to include a representation of torsion. One key feature of Maxwell's constructed models is that although they represent specific mechanisms that create the continuum-mechanical stresses, the inferences he made through them suppressed the specific causal mechanisms. In the reasoning context, Maxwell treated the specific mechanism of a model as representing the members of a class of mechanical system with that kind of causal relational structure. With hindsight we know that, in essence, Maxwell separated the notion of mechanical from the representation of "force" in electromagnetism, thereby providing for the first time in physics a mathematical representation of a nonmechanical, dynamical system. The models Maxwell's laws generate cannot be represented in the mechanical domains that served as the source domains in the construction of the models he used in deriving the equations.

Once identified, we can see that there are numerous examples of generic abstraction in conceptual innovation in science. In classical mechanics, for instance, Newton can be interpreted as using generic abstraction to reason about the commonalities among the motions of planets and of projectiles, and thus to formulate a unified mathematical representation of their motions. The models he used, such as drawn in figure 5.1, represent what is common among the members of specific classes of physical systems, viewed with respect to a problem context, in this case, projectiles and the moon. Newton's inverse-square representation of gravitation abstracts what a projectile and a planet have in common in the context of determining motion, for instance, that within the context of determining motion both can be represented as point masses. After Newton, the inverse-square-law model, then, served as a generic model of action-at-a-distance forces for those who tried to bring all forces into the scope of Newtonian mechanics—including, initially, electric and magnetic forces.

The kinds of abstractive processes we have been considering provide ways of selectively representing and reasoning with models. Idealization, limiting case, approximation, and generic abstraction provide a means of representing and integrating constraints stemming from different sources into models. Features not relevant to the problem solving can be instantiated in a model, possibly serving as scaffolding for the germane features. But to reason correctly by means of models requires recognizing which features are germane and which are cognitively inert within that problem-solving context.

6.2.3 Modes of Representing

The information one could bring to bear on a complex problem is considerable; thus the selectivity in representation afforded by focusing on specific constraints makes reasoning cognitively tractable. Throughout the analysis we have seen repeatedly that the choice of *how* to represent something is equally as important as *what* to represent for how effective a model is for reasoning. As discussed in chapter 4, different representational formats afford different kinds of manipulations, and so choice of format not only provides ways of being selective in the information represented, but also in kinds of inferences supported.

The exemplars furnish insights into ways in which imagistic representations in particular can provide advantages in dealing with representational problems leading to conceptual innovation. One possibility is that these formats recruit perceptual and motor processes in making inferences, such as inferring causality from the colocation of information in a diagram or inferring behavior through simulation of a mental model. On my interpretation of the S2 protocol, the open horizontal coil drawing (figure 3.12) has the distinctive and critical feature that it is in three-dimensional perspective. The shift in visual perspective is significant because the two-dimensional rod–spring models cannot represent the critical aspect of the behavior of a spring, that is, the mechanism of torsion. All subsequent renderings of the polygonal coil models are drawn with three-dimensional perspective. Although the information that the coil is three-dimensional could possibly have been conveyed in language or represented internally in propositional format, it is unlikely to have afforded the insight about torsion. For one thing, the propositional format would not exemplify the features that underlie it. For another, in S2's reasoning, the visualization represents not only the structure of the coil, but also its behavior. He understood the diagram to represent what David Gooding has called "a momentarily arrested process" (Gooding 2004, 211), that is, a dynamical object. The three-dimensional visual perspective affords a mental simulation—indicated by S2 drawing an arrow—in which the coil twists when pulled down. From this he inferred, through the steps we discussed, that torsion governs the stretch of a spring.

Another reason imagistic representation might be especially effective in conceptual innovation is that it can afford a means of bypassing constraints inherent in existing propositional or formulaic representations. When one is constructing and simulating a mental model, using imagistic representations might enable cognitive mechanisms to make novel connections that would be inhibited by, or not possible with, propositional or formulaic representations. Maxwell had the intuition that in seeking a mathematical representation of a novel domain, one needed to found the investigation on an embodied representation rather than begin from a purely formulaic representation. To paraphrase his argument, relying on purely mathematical representations runs the risk of being drawn to the analytical possibilities and subtleties of the mathematics and away from the phenomena. "Physical analogy" provides a way of selecting the aspects of the mathematics that are relevant to the target phenomena.

The contrast discussed earlier between Maxwell's method and Thomson's use of formal analogy is instructive. Transferring directly, for instance, Fourier's mathematical representation of heat to electrostatic phenomena, under appropriate substitutions, also carries over constraints inherent in a mathematical representation specific to phenomena not only similar to, but different from, the target phenomena. If inferences are made solely on the basis of manipulating the formulas, there is no way to capture and explore what might be different about—and possibly unique to—electromagnetism. Maxwell derived a mathematical representation from a model built first on the requirements of electromagnetism as thus far understood, which made it possible to represent the novel features of that domain. The models, themselves, provided constraints that led to new representational resources for the electromagnetic problem. As we saw, the implausibility of the vortex model as a mechanical system is suggested directly through simulating spinning vortices. Resolving the friction problem provided a way first of representing the causal relational structures between electricity and magnetism, and then of representing the relations among tensions and stresses associated with electrostatic phenomena—and so the energy components of the field, as we discussed.

Again, with hindsight, we can see that seeking a direct formal analogy with mathematical representations of solved problems in continuum mechanics (à la Thomson) could not work. Continuum mechanics does not have the resources to represent electromagnetism—a nonmechanical dynamical system. However, the mathematics of generalized dynamics— what today we call vector analysis and partial differential equations—does have that representational capacity. That is, mathematics can be applied to a wider range of phenomena than those falling in the scope of Newtonian mechanics. Using analogies as sources of constraints for building the intermediary models enabled Maxwell to use continuum mechanical knowledge in a highly selective manner, such that only those pieces consistent with the electromagnetic constraints were used. Once he derived an initial mathematical representation from the models, he and others could then take full advantage of the powerful representational capabilities of the mathematics to generalize, deepen, and extend the treatment of electromagnetism.

As with abstraction, knowing what to disregard in thinking with a particular representation is equally as important as knowing what to consider germane. In this, a particular visualization can have disadvantages as well as advantages. For one thing, if the reasoner does not have sufficient target information to know fully what to disregard, the model can be overgenerative, supporting inferences that do not apply to the target. The "lines of force" representation we discussed earlier that had a significant influence on the thinking of both Faraday and Maxwell provides a good instance.

Early in Faraday's research the diagram (figure 6.5) served to provide an abstract rendering of the patterns of iron filings surrounding a magnet. From the outset the image was intended as a two-dimensional representation of three-dimensional processes relating to a state of stress in the space surrounding the magnet. Faraday hypothesized that the configuration results from tensions along the lines and pressures among them. Later in the development of his field concept, however, he took the image to also

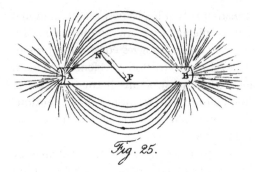

Figure 6.5
Faraday's drawing of the lines of force surrounding a magnet.

represent a dynamical model of the transmission and interconversion of forces, generally, through stresses and strains in, and various motions of, lines. Lines of force on this interpretation are substances through which all the forces of nature are transmitted, and matter is conceived as point centers of converging lines of force (Gooding 1981; Nersessian 1984a, 1985, 1992a; Tweney 1985). As I have discussed in detail in the works cited, the imagery is overgenerative in Faraday's reasoning. In general, the dynamical features of his broadest concept of field (what he called "physical lines," which is echoed in Maxwell's 1862–1862 paper title) originate in the kinds of motion possible for lines, such as bending, curving, and waving; rather than in continuous field processes. Further, the only explicit mathematical relation he formulated relates the induced force to the "number of lines" cut, but "number of" is a discrete measure (directly related to the lines), whereas a continuous measure is required for a field process.

Maxwell is one person who fully grasped Faraday's conception of forces (figure 6.6). As he vividly expressed in writing to Faraday: "You seem to see the lines of force curving round obstacles and driving plump at conductors, and swerving towards certain directions in crystals, and carrying with them everywhere the same amount of attractive power, spread wider or denser as the lines widen or contract" (Maxwell to Faraday, 9 November 1857, in Campbell and Garnett 1969, XV appendix). However, in Maxwell's mathematical analysis, the lines of force diagram came to be interpreted as representing states of stress and strain in the aetherial medium, through which the electromagnetic forces propagated continuously orthogonally to the lines rather than being transmitted along the lines. What Maxwell took from Faraday's interpretation were generic constraints of

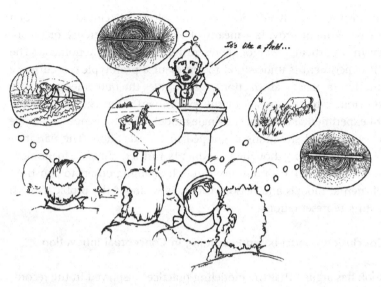

Figure 6.6
An imaginary lecture by Faraday. Where's Maxwell? (Drawing by Anne Larsen.)

tension and pressure, which provide the geometric constraints on shape of vortices. Iron filings placed in a magnetic field would assume the geometrical configuration in the sketch.

Finally, a critical dimension of model-based reasoning about physical systems is that the constructed models afford transformation through mental simulation. We have seen in the cognitive literature that simulation, more generally, is increasingly hypothesized to be constitutive of human cognition, where the human conceptual system is predicated on forms of reenactment. In reasoning processes, simulation can be understood as an epistemic endeavor, the purpose of which is to foster insight and inference through predicting future states of models and examining the consequences of these. In creating new states, simulative model-based reasoning takes advantage of the tacit information embedded in the constraints of a representation. As such, mental model simulation is a form of experimentation and lies on a continuum with full-blown thought experiments. As we saw, thought experiments provide ways of selectively bringing into comparison parts of conceptual structure. A conceptual structure systematically organizes concepts in relations with one another. Science stresses consistency and coherence, but a conceptual structure is rich and complex and it is unlikely that a person or a community could have a holistic grasp of it and its implications. The selective exemplifications of a thought experiment provide a means of exposing incoherence or inconsistency in a particular way of representing the target phenomena. The thought experiment is understood to represent a prototypical occurrence of a situation (a generic abstraction), which gives the outcomes generality and contributes to the impact of the experiment. That is, although the thought experimenter constructs a single model, its significance for a range of phenomena and situations is grasped in its execution. The narrative form of communicating thought experiments, further, can serve to promote conceptual change in a community through enabling others to construct parallel mental models and reason, themselves, about the problems with the existing representations.

6.3   Conclusion: Model-based Reasoning in Conceptual Innovation

This book has argued that the modeling practices displayed in the records of conceptual innovation and change in science need to be understood as forms of creative *reasoning*—in particular, that which creates candidate representations for processes of conceptual change. Embracing these as "methods" or "mechanisms" of conceptual innovation requires us to expand the traditional philosophical notions of reasoning. No claim is made that model-based reasoning is the only means of conceptual innovation. Although this analysis has focused on the initial construction of novel conceptual representations, model-based reasoning, too, can serve to transmit novel representations in a community. Of course, effecting conceptual change in science, as with all scientific change, involves other cognitive and sociocultural processes of the sort widely discussed in science studies. However, features of model-based reasoning discussed in this chapter—and developed throughout the book—make it a highly effective means of conceptual innovation.

   We have seen that analogical, imagistic, and simulative modeling enable selectively constructing mental models to satisfy constraints stemming from multiple sources. One significant function of analogies is to provide constraints for model-building in situations where the requisite resources are not available in a target domain. Imagistic representations facilitate perceptual inferences, provide a means of bypassing constraints in existing propositional and formulaic representations, and facilitate simulation processes. Dynamically manipulating the models in simulations affords inferences about the consequences of the interaction of explicit and tacit constraints. When conceptual innovation is cast in terms of processes of generating new and changing existing constraints, in the ways I have argued, model-based reasoning promotes conceptual change because it comprises effective ways of selectively abstracting, generating, and integrating constraints. Various abstractive processes facilitate integrating into mental models information that derives from more than one domain and information that might be represented in a variety of formats. These facilitate using—and in some instances, creating—mathematics to represent the phenomena. Among these, I have argued that generic abstraction is central to conceptual innovation in that, for retrieval, transfer, and integration to be possible, constraints need to be understood at a level of sufficient generality. It enables a kind of selectivity that restricts inferences to those that apply to members of a class of phenomena, not just the specific instantiation. Cycles of building, simulation, and inference can lead to the emergence of models that represent novel combinations of constraints, including the possibility of those that outstrip the representational resources of the specific domains from which the constraints were drawn—genuine conceptual innovations.

6.4 Reflexive Reflections: Wider Implications

Cognitive-historical analysis is a naturalistic method that seeks an integrative analysis, drawing from science studies, especially history of science and philosophy of science, and cognitive science. It is also reflexive and so, in concluding, I reflect briefly on some of the wider implications of my account of model-based reasoning for these fields. Rather than consider the implications per discipline, I select topics of interest that cut across them.

6.4.1 Learning
Learning in cognitive development and in science education are two areas where researchers have looked to accounts of conceptual change in science developed by historians and philosophers of science for insights. The premise underlying that research is that questions of how scientists construct accounts of phenomena that they do not yet have the concepts to express, how students learn concepts in science education, and how a child masters concepts he needs to acquire in the processes of cognitive development are all of a piece. This premise is proving a fertile supposition for framing research across these areas. Susan Carey (see Carey 2004 for an overview; Carey in press), in particular, argues that conceptual change in cognitive development employs bootstrapping mechanisms akin to those

of model-based reasoning as I have developed here. Cognitive development and science learning are entwined in the course of educating children and adolescents. On a "constructivist" view of learning, acquiring new concepts, as learning science demands, involves the active construction of the new representation (for an overview, see Duschl 1990). The continuum hypothesis leads to advancing the conjecture that the kinds of cognitive inquiry practices scientists use in creating concepts are directly relevant to the problem of how to assist students in learning the concepts of science.

The major lessons to be drawn for learning from the account of model-based reasoning developed here, which I have articulated on other occasions (see, e.g., Nersessian 1989, 1992c, 1995b) but are worth repeating, are as follows. First, conceptual innovation and change in science are— usually—incremental processes. That is, even when a creative insight might seem to occur in a sudden flash, it arises from prior modeling cycles: construction, manipulation, evaluation, and adaptation. Conceptual change in science and in mundane thinking is difficult. As with bootstrapping in science, models used in learning can provide stepping stones that incrementally take a learner through the steps necessary to acquiring scientific concepts and building scientific understanding. Second, model-based reasoning employs domain knowledge, knowledge of abstract domain-independent principles, and knowledge of how and when to use abstractions. Third, scientists' use of bootstrapping processes is explicit and metacognitively reflective. For the developing child and the science learner it is not. Rather than undermining the conjecture, this lesson can provide new research questions about the nature and development of metacognitive reflection in cognition, and suggest curriculum innovations to foster its development in learners.

Numerous model-based curricula innovations are underway (for a sample, see Clement and Steinberg 2002; Gilbert and Boulter 2000; Gobert and Buckley 2000; Justi and Gilbert 1999; Smith et al. 1997; Snir and Smith 1995; Wells, Hestenes, and Swackhamer 1995; Wiser 1995). Translating what we learn from model-based reasoning in scientific practice into effective strategies for learning in K–16 settings is not straightforward and opens numerous research questions. Among these are: What cognitive resources do children have from which to acquire the ability to engage in model-based reasoning, and what are the developmental trajectories of these resources? We know from the analogy research cited in chapter 4 that facility with analogy has a developmental trajectory. What about the ability to simulate mentally? To use diagrammatic representations? What about capacity for abstractive inference? In the K–8 curriculum, for instance, the kinds of models that will be effective will likely be quite different from those scientists would use. The point is that the kinds of reasoning processes should be model-based. The "dots-in-a-box" visual analogical models for teaching thermodynamics concepts provide excellent examples (see, e.g., Smith, Snir, and Grosslight 1992; Wiser 1995). Finally, given what I have said about the importance of the problem situation for model-based reasoning in science, an equally important set of issues arises with respect to this question: How can the contextual dimension of problem solving in science be translated into the contexts of learning environments? The cognitive-cultural systems of the classroom or instructional laboratory have their own unique constraints and affordances that will need to be figured into developing strategies for promoting learning through model-based reasoning.

6.4.2 Analogy

Thinking about analogy through the lens of modeling brings to the fore processes in need of explanation that are as yet unaccounted for in theories of analogy. As we saw in chapter 5, taking account of the creative work of constructing the models is central to understanding how analogy functioned to solve the representational problems. Current theories of analogy tend to focus on the retrieval of a source problem solution and subsequent mapping, and transfer. We saw that the progress made on understanding mapping and transfer is useful, especially in thinking about how to evaluate the "goodness" of an analogy. In creative use of analogy, though, where problems are ill defined (including problems that will require conceptual change), it often is the case that there is no existing source problem solution that affords a direct comparison. Rather, the comparison is indirect, requiring that the problem solver first construct the analog representation through which the corresponding target problem (or pieces of it) can be solved. In the cases we considered, the intermediary models are related to both the target and source domains, since they are built to satisfy constraints of both. Rather than transferring a mapping directly from the source, problems are solved in the intermediary models, and these provide the basis for the analogical mapping and transfer to the target. In effect, the model itself is treated as an analogical source. It is an object constructed to be related to the target in specific ways. The model provides enriched understandings of the target, leading to further iterations of model construction, possibly involving additional constraints from the same or additional analogical source domains.

The continuum hypothesis, bolstered by S2's spontaneous construction of intermediary models, leads to the conjecture that this kind of representation-building occurs fairly widely, and accounting for it is important for the theory of analogical reasoning. As far as I have been able to determine, there is scant empirical research directed at just how problem solvers build and modify their representations of targets and sources in analogical reasoning. Most research assumes a ready-to-hand analogical source solution, and that some relatively straightforward ways exist for modest re-representation of target or source when the match is not exact. I have purposely not discussed the computational models of analogy, since none of them is able to handle major facets of the way analogy is used in our exemplars. The primary focus of accounts in the AI literature is on mapping and transfer. Model construction might fall under what is called the problem of "re-representation," on which there is scant research but growing interest. Douglas Hofstadter and colleagues do make continual re-representations of the target and source in parallel with mapping and transfer processes (French 1995; Hofstadter 1995; Mitchell 1993). The LetterSpirit program, in particular, has led to conceptual innovation in creating novel font types, but such microworld approaches are unlikely to scale up to perform the kinds of model construction exhibited in our exemplars.[8]

Finally, we saw also that the analogies made use of imagistic and simulative processes, which some experimental findings also indicate. To accommodate these processes is going to require greater integration of research across various fields in cognitive science than is currently the case. In sum, then, my analysis points to the need for a richer, more nuanced account of analogy that addresses all dimensions.

6.4.3 Models and Modeling

There has been a recent explosion in research on models and modeling in science studies. These are now widely recognized as signature practices of the sciences—contemporary and past. This literature documents and analyzes various instances of model use in developing and using theories (see, e.g., Cartwright 1983; Giere 1988; Godfrey-Smith 2006; Magnani, Nersessian, and Thagard 1999; Morgan and Morrison 1999). Indeed, a significant segment of history and philosophy of science now gives models and modeling pride of place among scientific tools and practices. This shift of attention has come about not simply because of changes in the practices of scientists over time. Studies of past science provide ample evidence that although there are now new tools for enhancing and expanding these practices, since its inception, creating and thinking with models has been a standard part of problem solving in science. Rather, the shift has come about because many philosophers and historians no longer view science through the positivist lens of logic-based methods of inductive and hypothetico-deductive inference.

My analysis provides insight into scientists' use of models more generally. To date, research in the philosophical literature has tended to overemphasize the "realism" issue, at the expense of other important considerations about models; specifically, of the nature of the intellectual work that can be done through models and how a model functions to achieve scientific ends.[9] That focus seems a carry-over from earlier concerns about realism about theories, where models now are seen to "mediate between a theory and the world" (Morgan and Morrison 1999, 11). Models do provide the means for scientists to use theories and to examine their relation to phenomena, but they also use models in the absence of theories and as a means of constructing theories. The analysis of this book could be cast as coming at models from the other end: how scientists use models in discovery processes and to create theories. Viewed from the perspective of scientific discovery, models and modeling come first, with further analysis leading to formal expression in the laws and axioms of theories. Thus discovery provides another vantage point from which to consider how models conform to the world (Longino 2001), but it also brings to the fore issues about the nature of the reasoning done with models in problem solving. In particular, since models are constructed from and used as analogical sources in problem solving, it becomes imperative to have an understanding of analogical reasoning.

The account I have developed here synthesizes and expands upon my investigations of models as cognitive tools, in particular, of how scientists think and reason their way to novel conceptual representations by means of models. To figure out how models operate in this way requires looking carefully at details of exemplary cases of such use, and it requires thinking about the nature of the cognition that creates and makes use of such practices. Much of what I have said here about model-based reasoning can be extended beyond model use in conceptual change or a particular kind of modeling in physics, but specifically how will need to be determined by comparative examination. Model-based reasoning is widely employed as a problem-solving tool across the sciences, and uses share features even when carried out in different domains. Analogical or visual processes in modeling in physics, for example, will function much the same as analogical or visual processes in modeling in biology. There are more kinds of modeling than considered here, such as statistical modeling in psychology or computational modeling in physics, that this analysis says nothing about. I leave it to those working in other domains and with different kinds of models to determine what of my account will carry over. However, from other research I have been conducting on physical models constructed for the purposes of *in vitro* experimentation and computational simulation models in the areas of tissue engineering, neural engineering, and bio-robotics, the kind of modeling practices examined in this book appear to belong to a kind of model use that might be called "discovery through construction" (Nersessian 2005; Nersessian et al. 2003). In the process of constructing and manipulating models—mental, physical, computational surrogates—scientists gain novel insight and provisional understanding of aspects of target phenomena. Through these practices science makes progress in a domain in the absence of what is customarily understood as "knowledge."

My own further research into model-based reasoning practices has been examining how researchers in laboratories in biomedical engineering and bio-robotics create and use *in vitro* physical and computational models to simulate *in vivo* phenomena on which they cannot experiment directly. I have chosen these kinds of laboratories for several reasons, all relating to my objective of creating an account in which cognition and culture are mutually implicative in the modeling practices of innovative research. First, it is widely known that creative outcomes often arise from bringing together insights from disparate sources. Interdisciplinary research laboratories provide settings where novel achievements can arise from approaching problems in ways that force together concepts, methods, discourses, artifacts, and epistemologies of two or more disciplines. Second, these particular laboratories are sites of learning that aim to create researchers who are in themselves interdisciplinary individuals, rather than disciplinary contributors to an interdisciplinary team. Third, numerous studies of research laboratories conducted by sociologists and anthropologists have shown the fruitfulness of studying research laboratories and groups for thinking about the cultures of science, but scarcely any research has looked at cognitive practices (see Dunbar 1995 for an exception) or with the problem of integration in mind. My research group approaches the laboratory studies from the environmental perspective in cognitive science (discussed briefly in chapter 1), which casts human cognition, generally, as occurring in complex systems situated in social, cultural, and material environments. With the objective of interpretive integration, the trick is to create accounts that are neither primarily cognitive with culture tacked on nor the reverse, and this requires rethinking current interpretive categories. I provide one brief example. In the tissue engineering laboratory, where the overarching problem is to create living vascular substitutes for implanting in humans, researchers construct technological artifacts in order to perform *in vitro* simulations of current models of *in vivo* biological processes in human arteries. These perform as what they call "model systems"—locales where engineered artifacts interface with living cell cultures—in specific problem-solving processes. These artifacts are what cultural studies of science refer to as the "material culture" of the community, but they also function as what cognitive studies of science refer to as "cognitive artifacts" participating in the reasoning and representational processes of a distributed cognitive system. My point is that within the research of the laboratories, they are both, and it is not possible to fathom how they produce knowledge by focusing exclusively on one or the other aspect. They are representations of current understandings and thus play a role in model-based and simulative reasoning; they are central to social practices related to community membership; they are sites of learning; they provide ties that bind one generation of researchers (around five years) to another; they perform as cultural "ratchets" that enable one generation to build upon the results of the previous, and thus move the problem solving forward. In sum, they are central in the cultural-cognitive fabric in which scientific creativity is nurtured and can flourish. Problem solving with devices (simulation models) requires that researchers merge concepts, models, and methods of biology and engineering. The model-systems need to be understood not just as "boundary objects" (Star and Griesemer 1989) existing in the "trading zones" (Galison 1997) of two or more communities and as mediating communication, but as sites of interdisciplinary melding of concepts, models, methods, artifacts, and epistemologies—where genuine novelty emerges.

Notes

1 Creativity in Conceptual Change: A Cognitive-Historical Approach

1. The notion of scientific change as a problem-solving process, in fact, cuts across work in history, philosophy, and psychology as practiced in Europe early in the last century. That notion is represented in the work of various psychologists of the Würtzburg and Gestalt schools and of Jean Piaget; of a founder of cognitive science, Herbert Simon, who traced this facet of his intellectual lineage to a psychologist of the Würtzburg school, Otto Selz; of the historians Emil Meyerson and Alexandre Koyré; and of the philosopher Karl Popper, also influenced by the Würtzburg school. There was considerable influence among these strains of thought. William Berkson and John Wettersten (1984) provide a brief account of the relation of the Würtzburg school to Popper's philosophy of science, which indicates that there is a fascinating piece of intellectual history on this topic in need of a fuller treatment.

2. As especially notable examples, see Andersen, Barker, and Chen 2006; Darden 1980, 1991; Gentner et al. 1997; Giere 1988, 1992, 1994; Gooding 1990; Griesemer 1991a,b; Griesemer and Wimsatt 1989; Holmes 1981, 1985; Rudwick 1976; Shelley 1996; Spranzi 2004; Thagard 1992; Trumpler 1997; Tweney 1987, 1992.

3. Several philosophers of science did take analogy in science as a serious topic of discussion even in the heyday of positivism. For Max Black (1962), Norman Campbell (1920), and Mary Hesse (1963), analogy serves an explanatory function and provides some basis for hypothesis generation. Further, they held that analogy is constitutive of theories in that analogies continue to provide meaning for new theoretical terms and act as a basis for elaboration and extension of a theory. But they did not develop theories of analogy adequate to address the problem of explaining how it could generate novel concepts. On the positivist side, in Rudolph Carnap's *Logical Foundations of Probability* (1950), analogy occupies just a single page in the Appendix. He concludes that "reasoning by analogy, although admissible, can usually yield only weak results" (569). I have been arguing that science provides ample evidence of productive, creative reasoning by analogy that establishes it as yielding powerful results. The way to resolve the discrepancy is to understand that

reasoning by analogy is not only argument, but also modeling. Black, Campbell, and Hesse made some linkage between models and analogies, but did not explicate how model representations and reasoning with models differ from those used in argument.

4. I owe this observation to Abner Shimony in private correspondence.

2   Model-based Reasoning Practices: Historical Exemplar

1. I disagree, however, with his claim (Siegel 1991, 75) that Maxwell was prevented initially from making the vortices elastic since "Thomson saw elasticity as resulting from motion in a mechanical substratum." The vortices are a form of motion in a mechanical substratum in the model and, as noted earlier, elasticity is consistent with the analysis in Part I. A more likely reason is that Maxwell had considered and rejected this alternative in carrying out the calculation in Part II and was reluctant to modify the specific features of the vortex–idle wheel version of the model.

2. See also Chalmers 1986, which argues in response to my analyses (Nersessian 1984a,b) to the contrary that the models were an "unproductive digression."

3. William Berkson also criticizes the symmetry argument as presented by Jackson (Berkson 1974, 338–339).

4. A few commentators at the time I first encountered Maxwell's work did take seriously at least parts of the analogy, most significantly Joan Bromberg (Bromberg 1968) whose analysis of the displacement current I found useful and Berkson (1974), whose work I found useful for my later thinking about problem situations. Later, Siegel (Siegel 1991, 1986) presented arguments in favor of the centrality of the analogical model in the 1861–1862 paper. Mary Hesse's position is more difficult to characterize because she did see analogy as playing a significant role in hypothesis formation and theory interpretation in general. However, it is puzzling that her analysis (Hesse 1973) of Maxwell's theory passes over the 1861–1862 paper—what I am arguing contains the main generative work.

5. "If you want to find out anything from the theoretical physicists about the methods they use, I advise you to stick closely to one principle: don't listen to their words, fix your attention on their deeds. To him who is a discoverer in this field, the products of his imagination appear so necessary and natural that he regards them, and would like to have them regarded by others, not as creations of thought but as given realities" (Einstein 1973, 264).

3   Model-based Reasoning Practices: Protocol Study Exemplar

1. The coding was developed in detail in related work with my former graduate student, Todd Griffith, and his coadvisor, my colleague, Ashok Goel. That research created a computational model of the reasoning processes, and the coding formal-

ism was related specifically to Goel's computational reasoning methods, such as "model-based analogy" and "structure-based model transformation" (see Griffith 1999).

2. I am indebted to John Clement's generosity in giving me the transcripts of this protocol, and the entire set of protocols for the computational analysis by Todd Griffith. I greatly appreciate the many discussions we have had of this material over the years and the comments he contributed to the final version of this chapter. Further, I appreciate and acknowledge the discussions with James Greeno several years ago as I first wrestled with this material and how it compares with the Maxwell case, when I enjoyed the hospitality of his guest house and of Noreen Greeno. Finally, my analysis has profited from numerous discussions with Todd Griffith and Ashok Goel in developing a computational analysis of model-based reasoning in the entire set of protocols collected by Clement.

3. As transcribed, the protocol consists of twenty-two pages and seven sheets of S2's original sketches. Each number refers to a continuous utterance by either the subject or the interviewer, in sequence, as marked in the transcript. So, for instance, "005" refers to the fifth utterance during the course of the problem solving session. Dashes indicate pauses.

4. Griffith (1999) argues that it is equally plausible that given experience he retrieved the model by searching his memory for an analogue to "stretchable, wire-like things." This interpretation works better with the computational constraints of Griffith's analysis, but I consider it not as likely an interpretation. Additional evidence for the simulation interpretation appears later (007) *"I'm still led back to this notion . . . of a spring straightened out"* and (009) where the rod is first referred to as *"the unwound spring."* Further, S2 continued to refer to the rod as an "unwound," "stretched," or "uncoiled" spring throughout the protocol.

5. Clement (1988) found evidence that in a sample of ten experts who worked on the spring problem, a large majority of the thirty-one germane analogies that were generated for the problem were created via transformations rather than by associations to similar features. He has also hypothesized that conserving transformations can be used to evaluate the soundness of an already generated analogy (Clement 2004).

4 The Cognitive Basis of Model-based Reasoning Practices: Mental Modeling

1. I thank Margriet van der Heijden for giving me her transcription of this section of the interview and permission to use it.

2. Although I am not drawing on his work here, the *locus classicus* for the introduction of the notion of "iconic" as a way in which representations refer to objects is C. S. Pierce (1931–1935): "An *Icon* is a sign which refers to the Object that it denotes merely by virtue of characters of its own, and which it possesses, just the same,

whether any such Object actually exists or not. It is true that unless there really is such an Object, the Icon does not act as a sign; but this has nothing to do with its character as a sign. Anything whatever, be it quality, existent individual, or law, is an Icon of anything, in so far as it is like that thing and used as a sign of it" (*Collected Papers* II, 247).

3. Holland et al. (1986) do develop an account of mental modeling that includes causal reasoning. However, since in this work I focus on accounts supporting iconic mental models, I will not discuss their account of propositional models.

4. Recent computational modeling work on the origin of representations shows that internal representational structures can emerge in reactive creatures (creatures that just sense and act—they do no internal processing) and such internal structures would "encapsulate" actions, and thus support simulation. (Chandrasekharan and Stewart 2007).

5. This interpretation receives additional support from the formal analysis conducted by Barwise and Etchemendy (1995).

6. The ability to mentally animate is highly correlated with scores on tests of spatial ability (Hegarty and Sims 1994). However, as Mary Hegarty also stresses, the mental representations underlying animation need not be what are customarily thought of as "mental images." Images are often taken to be vivid and detailed holistic representations, such as those in a photograph or a movie, where simulation would take place all at once. However, the imagery literature supports the notion that imagery most often is largely sketchy and schematic and that animation of an image can be piecemeal, as supported by Hegarty's research. Kosslyn's highly elaborated neuroscience account of imagery (Kosslyn 1994) argues that transformations of the image most likely take place outside of the visual buffer through connections with long-term memory representations, with the image in the buffer being "refreshed" with the updated transformation.

5 Representation and Reasoning: Analogy, Imagery, Thought Experiment

1. A scattering of psychological studies do point to the possibility of a visual dimension to some analogy use (see, e.g., Beveridge and Parkins 1987; Catrambone, Craig, and Nersessian 2006; Craig, Nersessian, and Catrambone 2002a,b). There have been some computational analyses of visual aspects of analogy (see, e.g., Croft and Thagard 2002; Davies 2004; Davies, Nersessian, and Goel 2002; Ferguson 1994; Hofstadter 1995; Thagard, Gochfield, and Hardy 1992; Yaner 2007).

2. This often repeated attribution is in fact not historically accurate. There is no evidence that Rutherford ever used the solar system–atom analogy as presented in the analogy literature, and there are no discussions or drawings of it anywhere in his published or unpublished work. There is an interesting twist, though. There is some indication that when Rutherford was thinking about whether the force of

nucleus on the alpha particles was attractive or repulsive, he consulted Newton's analysis of the hyperbola and the inverse-square law. David Wilson (1983) has noted that Rutherford's copy of the *Principia* contains undated marginal notes at the section where Newton presents his analysis, which was used in formulating the law of universal gravitation. However, this analysis was of forces in a *generic* situation where there was a central body and another body in orbit around it; that is, not specifically the solar system, and not only attractive forces. So there might indeed be some connection between the solar system model and Rutherford's model of the atom, but not as customarily understood.

3. Marta Spranzi (2004) shows that Galileo, too, used analogies to create what I am calling "intermediary hybrid models" from those analogies in his analysis of the possibility of mountains on the moon. Clement (1989) has remarked on what he calls S2's "bridging analogies" but he does not address specifically how the intermediary models are hybrid representations embedding target and source constraints, as I have laid out in chapter 3.

4. I believe it was Paul Thagard who used this comparison in a lecture I heard.

5. Both Max Black (1962) and Wilfrid Sellars (1973), although not commenting on any historical case, argue that the mapping of relational structure as opposed to objects and properties would be central to creative analogies. Sellars makes this point in a dispute with Mary Hesse whose theory of analogy tries to account for mapping more in terms of properties than of relational structure. Indeed, Hesse and also Peter Achinstein discuss Maxwell's work and do take his use of analogy seriously. However, without the emphasis on mapping relational structure they are unable to account satisfactorily for its productivity. I suspect her focus on properties is the reason why Hesse, who did substantial work on Maxwell, overlooked the importance of the analysis in his second paper (Maxwell 1861–1862)—the one on which I focus here. She began with the third paper (Maxwell 1864), in which, once he knew how to represent the electromagnetic general dynamical quantities, he rederived the equations mainly from electromagnetic considerations. But as I have argued it was only through reasoning with the analogical models in the second paper that he knew how to represent these in general dynamical terms.

6. I am limiting my discussion to psychological research and am not discussing computational implementations. Although these implementations are often the means through which competing interpretations of the psychological evidence are investigated, they also make implementation assumptions to fit the kinds of computational tools employed. For our purposes we need not delve into the details and the differences of how the computational models carry out the inferential processes, and which might be better for what reasons. They all are successful at producing outcomes that are consistent with a range of observed behaviors, but the psychological theories on which they are based make competing claims, so clearly analogy is still an area in need of further investigation.

7. There is an ongoing controversy around representation building concerning the cognitive theories as they are implemented as computational models. Douglas Hofstadter argued from his broad study of spontaneous creative analogies, especially by scientists, and his investigations of analogical processes in AI "micro-worlds," that conceptual information plays a significant role in analogical mapping. He argues that creating the source representation to use in mapping is a critical process for understanding analogical reasoning (Hofstadter 1995). In providing the program with pared-down representations constructed by the modeler, as done by the programs at that time, the researchers are doing much of the creative work, rather than the model. In response, Forbus, Gentner, and Law (1995) argued that domain knowledge is needed for such representation-building and to include this would make the use of analogy a domain-specific process. This conclusion, however, does not follow. Whatever the domain, the same underlying cognitive processes can be at work in modifying or constructing representations, extracting relational structure, making and transferring candidate inferences, and making evaluations along the way. That is, the analogical processes, though drawing on domain knowledge, are themselves domain general. They admit that representation building might be "interleaved" with analogical processes, but they claim that this is not part of analogy per se. "Analogy" is to be understood in terms of its core processes of mapping and transfer, which on their account are purely syntactical. However, what is at issue here is more significant than terminology. Following that debate, Forbus and Gentner have modified their system to construct the initial representations used in analogy and have moved to an "incremental" mapping process that dynamically adjusts the mapping on the basis of new information from the target. However, the target and sources are not re-represented in these processes, and the kind of intermediary model representations we are discussing are not considered at all. I will say a bit more about Hofstadter's approach in chapter 6.

8. I am indebted to Catherine Elgin for leading me to see the importance of exemplification and its relation to the notion of "same kind as" I have been arguing is an evaluation criterion in model-based reasoning; for sharing her recent unpublished work on the topic with me; and for the wonderful lunch conversations while I was at Radcliffe Institute.

9. I thank Andrea Woody for reminding me of this facet of Goodman's account of representation in her APA commentary on my symposium paper on analogy.

10. Unlike in the case of S2, we cannot be sure that Maxwell drew diagrams while reasoning. Several factors enter into my judgment that he is likely to have done so, including that: (1) he repeatedly noted the importance of making mathematical relations visual; (2) there are drawings in other draft materials; and (3) he used drawings in communicative activities. Although no draft materials related to this episode exist, in drafts of other papers and in letters where he discussed his developing ideas, he did make such drawings. As I have argued elsewhere (Nersessian 1984a, 1992a, 2002c), there is sufficient evidence to support the position that the reasoning in the published paper is reasonably faithful to Maxwell's own reasoning processes.

We can look at him as leading his audience through his own reasoning processes as a rhetorical move to help his colleagues to construct corresponding mental models through which to understand the new field representation.

Further, because the analysis in chapter 2 is based on historical records, it might give the impression that the relation between mental modeling and representing is asynchronous, with, for instance, the models preceding the equations. As with S2 and the analysis in chapter 4, my hypothesis is that for Maxwell, too, mental modeling and representing are interactive.

11. Gradually since the 1980s, the situation in science studies has changed from one where visual representations are largely neglected to one where accounts of the use of visual representation detailing specific and quite varied usages are too numerous to survey. An early study that still provides a model for examining the interaction of cultural and cognitive aspects of visual representation is that by Martin Rudwick (1976) on how visual representation revolutionized geological thinking and practice. He argued that the development of geology as a science involved learning how and what features to abstract and represent in visual formats that could be used both in analysis and in communication. One significant invention was the "ideal section" that represents spatial relations among different classes of rocks and the interpretation of these in temporal and causal terms, thus implicitly displaying and conveying theoretical assumptions (Rudwick 1976, 166). Rudwick argued that in modern geological practice sections function like thought experiments in that a tract is imagined as if it were sliced vertically and opened like an "artificial cliff" (ibid., 164). His analysis both connected the development of several salient modes of representation to changes in practice and advanced the view that in order to give an adequate historical explanation for how the development of modes of representation change scientific practices, one needs to understand the cognitive functions of visual representation in mundane thought.

12. Whether Maxwell experienced mental imagery can only be speculated about. His writings are peppered with talk of "mental operations" related to visualization in physical and mathematical reasoning that would lead speculation in the direction of an affirmative answer. In addition, the comments he made on the need for *physical* analogies lead in that direction. One particularly nice expression of his thoughts about embodying mathematics for reasoning purposes appears in an article he wrote for the Cambridge Philosophical Society about the Lagrangian notion of a connected system:

In the present day it is necessary for physical inquirers to obtain clear ideas in dynamics that they may be able to study dynamical theories of the physical sciences. We must therefore avail ourselves of the labours of the mathematicians, and selecting from his symbols those which correspond to physical quantities, we must retranslate them into the language of dynamics. In this way our words will call up the mental image, not of certain operations of the calculus, but of certain characteristics of the motion of bodies. (Maxwell 1876, 308)

Another equally vivid expression appears in an article written for *Nature* about the new mathematical formalism, the method of quaternions, that he employed in the *Treatise*: "It [the method] does not . . . encourage the hope that mathematicians may give their minds a holiday, by transferring all their work to their pens. It calls upon us at every step to form a mental image of the geometrical features represented by the symbols, so that in studying geometry by this method we have our minds engaged with geometrical ideas, and are not permitted to fancy ourselves geometers when we are only arithmeticians" (Maxwell 1873, 137).

13. Another piece of the interview with Terrance Tao used as an epigraph to chapter 4 is interesting in this context. Interviewer: "You seem to visualize all these problems?" Tao: "It's funny because when I was a child I was actually very bad at visualising things. I remember that someone gave me this intelligence test and there was this shape, this visual shape, and the question was if it could correspond to another shape, and I couldn't do that. I could not visualise complicated objects. I can do that now because, well, I do it more abstract and put like letters in the corners and see how the letters connect to each other."

14. Figuring out the interface between conducting and dielectric media given the model was a complex problem, and that was likely the reason for the time delay between the solutions of the problems of electromagnetic and electrostatic induction. The solution was to make the vortices elastic, although they had been treated as rigid in the earlier calculations. For a full treatment of this issue see Nersessian (2002a,c) and Siegel (1991).

15. Nenad Miščević (Miščević 1992) argued independently in the same year in favor of a mental modeling account of thought experimenting.

16. Sociologists of science have pointed out that the form of real-world experimental narratives has been crafted by scientists and has changed over time. Early narratives were much more richly detailed than is now customary (Dear 1985; Shapin 1984). Steven Shapin claims these narrative forms provide a "literary technology" (Shapin 1984, 194), developed to establish the practice of communicating experimental results in the absence of the experiment. He claims that the style of Robert Boyle's experimental narratives reflects the circumstances that Boyle sought to gain authority for the experimental method through enabling the reader to be a "virtual witness" of the experiment. The narratives create an "impression of verisimilitude" that Shapin claims conveys authority and compels assent. On a mental modeling account, a significant reason why Boyle's narratives were effective rhetorical devices is that the narratives functioned to assist the reader in constructing a mental simulation that enabled them to understand the outcome that they did not actually witness themselves. In contrast, Larry Holmes (Holmes 1990) has pointed out that the experimental narratives produced by the members of the Académie des Sciences during the same historical period are much more succinct and quite similar to those in the modern scientific literature. He argues that this stems, in part, from the

practice of French Academicians of carrying out communal investigations, so authority was not in question. In this case, the expertise of the group can be assumed in conveying results. On my view, where there is a highly developed community of experimental practitioners, a more succinct experimental narrative will be effective, since community understanding about procedures and apparatus can be presumed as part of what the community of readers will interpolate into their mental models of the experiment.

6 Creativity in Conceptual Change

1. I would, of course, prefer that he had titled his book *The Processes of Creation*.

2. So, on my account, "normal" and "revolutionary" science are not marked by different methods, but by the nature of the problems and problem situations in which the methods are used.

3. See Thagard 1992 for an extended discussion of the nature and function of concepts in cognitive science and philosophy of science.

4. Whether an analogy is a "near" or "distant" analogy (see, e.g., Dunbar 1995, 2000) needs to be understood as relative to the problem situation in which it is made, and not from our own perspective. From our perspective, for instance, Maxwell's analogy between electromagnetism and continuum mechanics seems a "distant" analogy, but his community considered that electromagnetic phenomena were possibly a kind of continuum phenomena. So, too, the "generic" atom–solar system analogy we discussed in chapter 5, note 2 can be seen as a "near" analogy in its problem situation. Rutherford in his context of considering the nature of the forces of the nucleus on alpha particles is likely to have drawn on Newton's generic analysis of forces Rutherford thought to be of that kind.

5. See Nersessian 1984a, 1985, 2001 for a meaning schema format that draws from prototype and frame views; Andersen, Barker, and Chen 2006 for an extended analysis of conceptual change in scientific revolutions using Barsalou's dynamic frames; and Giere 1992 for similar use of Lakoff's idealized cognitive models.

6. Wonderful pictures and audio recordings of this bird can be found by searching on "screamer" at the website of the Cornell Lab of Ornithology, Macaulay Library Sound and Video Catalog: www.animalbehaviorarchive.org.

7. Since developing the notion of "generic" abstraction to address the issue of the generality of inferences from a specific model, I have discovered it has an old history in empiricist philosophy. Berkeley, for example, argues contra Locke that in reasoning about a triangle, one must construct a specific representation ("idea") of a particular triangle. The mind, however, has the ability to understand and grasp the general in the particular, for example, what inferences are common to all kinds of triangle (Berkeley 1968, introduction, sections 4–19).

8. A point with which Hofstadter concurred in a conversation we had about this issue in January 2005.

9. One can accept and make use of the insights and results developed in my analysis while remaining agnostic on the realism–antirealism debate, as Arabatzis (2006) claims for his "biography"of the electron. There are aspects of model construction that speak to either side. As representations, scientific models are built, partially, on empirical constraints stemming from confirmed experimental results. This provides an argument against an "anything goes" version of social constructivism. But the models also knowingly instantiate unrealistic features. In this analysis I have chosen to focus on another, more neglected, dimension of modeling in science about which something definite can be said: the nature of the reasoning carried out through modeling. Arabatzis also argues that the issues of realism and rationality have often been conflated in postpositivist discussions of representational change, and he admonishes that they be separated. The analysis I have developed here provides strong support for the rationality of such change.

References

Allwein, G., and J. Barwise (1996). *Logical Reasoning with Diagrams*. New York: Oxford University Press.

Andersen, H., P. Barker, and X. Chen (2006). *The Cognitive Structure of Scientific Revolutions*. Cambridge: Cambridge University Press.

Andersen, H., X. Chen, and P. Barker (1996). "Kuhn's mature philosophy of science and cognitive psychology." *Philosophical Psychology* 9: 347–363.

Andersen, H., and N. J. Nersessian (2000). "Nomic concepts, frames, and conceptual change." *Philosophy of Science* 67: s234–241.

Arabatzis, T. (2006). *Representing Electrons: A Biographical Approach to Theoretical Entities*. Chicago: University of Chicago Press.

Arditi, A., J. D. Holtzman, and S. M. Kosslyn (1988). "Mental imagery and sensory experience in congenital blindness." *Neuropsychologia* 26: 1–12.

Barsalou, L. W. (1999). "Perceptual Symbol Systems." *Behavioral and Brain Sciences* 22: 577–609.

Barsalou, L. W. (2003). "Situated simulation in the human conceptual system." *Language and Cognitive Processes* 18: 513–562.

Barsalou, L. W., and J. J. Prinz (1997). "Mundane creativity in perceptual symbol systems." In *Creative Thought: A Investigation of Conceptual Structures and Processes*, ed. T. Ward, S. M. Smith, and J. Vaid, 267–307. Washington, D.C., American Psychological Association.

Barsalou, L. W., W. K. Simmons, A. K. Barby, and C. D. Wilson (2003). "Grounding conceptual knowledge in modality-specific systems." *Trends in Cognitive Science* 7: 84–91.

Barsalou, L. W., K. O. Solomon, and L. L. Wu (1999). "Perceptual simulation in conceptual tasks." In *Cultural, Typological, and Psychological Perspectives in Cognitive Linguistics: The Proceedings of the Fourth Annual Conference of the International Cognitive

Linguistics Association, 3: 209–228, ed. M. K. Hiraga, C. Sinha, and S. Wilcox. Amsterdam: John Benjamins.

Bauer, M. I., and P. N. Johnson-Laird (1993). "How diagrams can improve reading." *Psychological Science* 4: 372–378.

Barwise, J., and J. Etchemendy (1995). "Heterogenous Logic." In *Diagrammatic Reasoning: Cognitive and Computational Perspectives,* 211–234, ed. J. Glasgow, N. H. Narayanan, and B. Chandrasekaran. Cambridge, Mass.: MIT Press.

Bell, V. A., and P. N. Johnson-Laird (1998). "A model theory of modal reasoning." *Cognitive Science* 22 (1): 25–51.

Bergen, B., Chang, N., and S. Narayan (2004). *Simulated Action in an Embodied Construction Grammar.* Proceedings of the 26th Annual Meeting of the Cognitive Science Society, Chicago. Hillsdale, N.J.: Lawrence Erlbaum.

Berkeley, G. (1968). *A Treatise Concerning the Principles of Human Knowledge.* In *British Empiricist Philosophers,* 163–178, ed. A. J. Ayer and R. Winch. New York: Simon and Schuster.

Berkson, W. (1974). *Fields of Force: The Development of a World View from Faraday to Einstein.* New York: John Wiley.

Berkson, W., and J. Wettersten (1984). *Learning from Error: Karl Popper's Psychology of Learning.* LaSalle, Ill.: Open Court.

Beveridge, M., and E. Parkins (1987). "Visual representation in analogical problem solving." *Memory and Cognition* 15: 230–237.

Black, M. (1962). *Models and Metaphors.* Ithaca: Cornell University Press.

Blanchette, I., and K. Dunbar (2000). "How analogies are generated: The roles of structural and superficial similarity." *Memory and Cognition* 28: 108–124.

Bobrow, D. G. (ed.) (1985). *Qualitative Reasoning about Physical Systems.* Cambridge, Mass.: MIT Press.

Boden, M. A. (1990). *The Creative Mind: Myths and Mechanisms.* New York: Basic Books.

Brass, M., H. Bekkering, and W. Prinz (2002). "Movement observation affects movement execution in a simple response task." *Acta Psychologica* 106.

Brass, M., and C. Heyes (2005). "Imitation: Is cognitive neuroscience solving the correspondence problem?" *Trends in Cognitive Science* 9: 489–495.

Bromberg, J. (1968). "Maxwell's displacement current and his theory of light." *Archive for History of Exact Science* 4: 218–234.

Brown, J. S., A. Collins, and P. Duguid (1989). "Situated cognition and the culture of learning." *Educational Researcher* 18: 32–42.

Bryant, D. J., and B. Tversky (1999). "Mental representations of perspective and spatial relations from diagrams and models." *Journal of Experimental Psychology: Learning, Memory, and Cognition* 25: 137–156.

Bryant, D. J., B. Tversky, and N. Franklin (1992). "Internal and external spatial frameworks for representing described scenes." *Journal of Memory and Language* 31: 74–98.

Buchwald, J. Z. (1985). *From Maxwell to Microphysics*. Chicago: University of Chicago Press.

Campbell, N. R. (1920). *Physics, the Elements*. Cambridge: Cambridge University Press.

Campbell, L., and W. Garnett (1969). *The Life of James Clerk Maxwell (with a new preface and appendix with letters by Robert H. Kargon)*. New York: Johnson Reprint Corp.

Carey, S. (1985). *Conceptual Change in Childhood*. Cambridge, Mass.: MIT Press.

Carey, S. (2004). "Bootstrapping and the origin of concepts." *Daedalus* (winter): 59–68.

Carey, S. (in press). *The Origin of Concepts*. London: Oxford University Press.

Carnap, R. (1936). "Testability and meaning." *Philosophy of Science* 3: 401–467.

Carnap, R. (1950). *Logical Foundations of Probability*. Chicago, Ill.: University of Chicago Press.

Cartwright, N. (1983). *How the Laws of Physics Lie*. Oxford: Clarendon Press.

Catrambone, R., D. L. Craig, and N. J. Nersessian (2006). "The role of perceptually represented structure in analogical problem solving." *Memory and Cognition* 34: 1126–1134.

Chalmers, A. F. (1973). "Maxwell's methodology and his application of it to electromagnetism." *Studies in the History and Philosophy of Science* 4 (2): 107–164.

Chalmers, A. F. (1986). "The heuristic role of Maxwell's mechanical model of electromagnetic phenomena." *Studies in the History and Philosophy of Science* 17: 415–427.

Chambers, D., and D. Reisberg (1985). "Can mental images be ambiguous?" *Journal of Experimental Psychology: Human Perception and Performance* 11 (3): 317–328.

Chandrasekaran, B. (2005). "What makes a bunch of marks a diagrammatic representation, and another bunch a sentential representation?" In *Proceedings of the AAAI Spring Symposium, Reasoning with Mental and External Diagrams: Computational Modeling and Spatial Assistance*, ed. T. Barakowsky, C. Freksa, M. Hegarty, and R. Lowe. Menlo Park, Calif.: AAAI Press.

Chandrasekaran, B., J. I. Glasgow, and N. H. Narayanan (1995). "An introduction to diagrammatic reasoning." In *Diagrammatic Reasoning: Cognitive and Computational Perspectives,* ed. J. I. Glasgow, N. H. Narayanan, and B. Chandrasekaran. Menlo Park, Calif.: AAAI Press: xv–xxviii.

Chandrasekharan, S., and T. C. Stewart (2007). "The origin of epistemic structures and proto-representations." *Adaptive Behaviour* 15: 329–353.

Cheng, P. C.-H. (1999a). "Unlocking conceptual learning in mathematics and science with effective representational systems." *Computers in Education* 33 (2–3): 109–130.

Cheng, P. C.-H. (1999b). "Representational analysis and design: What makes an effective representation for learning probability theory?" Technical Report No. 65. Centre for Research and Development, Instruction, and Training. University of Sussex, Brighton, UK.

Cheng, P. C.-H., R. Lowe, and M. Scaife (2001). "Cognitive science approaches to understanding diagrammatic representations." *Artificial Intelligence Review* 15: 5–27.

Cheng, P. C.-H., and H. A. Simon (1995). "Scientific discovery and creative reasoning with diagrams." In *The Creative Cognition Approach,* ed. T. W. a. R. Finke. Cambridge, Mass.: MIT Press.

Chi, M. T. H. (1997). "Quantifying qualitative analyses of verbal data: A practical guide." *Journal of the Learning Sciences* 6 (3): 271–315.

Chi, M. T. H., P. J. Feltovich, and R. Glaser (1981). "Categorization and representation of physics problems by experts and novices." *Cognitive Science* 5: 121–152.

Clancey, W. J. (1997). *Situated Cognition: On Human Knowledge and Computer Representations.* Cambridge: Cambridge University Press.

Clement, J. (1986). *Methods Used to Evaluate the Validity of Hypothesized Analogies.* Proceedings of the Ninth Annual Meeting of the Cognitive Science Society. Hillsdale, N.J.: Lawrence Erlbaum.

Clement, J. (1988). "Observed methods for generating analogies in scientific problem solving." *Cognitive Science* 12 (4): 563–586.

Clement, J. (1989). "Learning via model construction and criticism." In *Handbook of Creativity: Assessment, Theory, and Research,* 341–381, ed. G. Glover, R. Ronning, and C. Reynolds. New York: Plenum.

Clement, J. (1994). "Use of physical intuition and imagistic simulation in expert problem solving." In *Implicit and Explicit Knowledge,* 204–242, ed. D. Tirosh. Norwood, N.J.: Ablex Publishing.

Clement, J. (2003). "Imagistic simulation in scientific model construction." In *Proceedings of the Cognitive Science Society 25*, 258–263, ed. D. Alterman and D. Kirsch. Hillsdale, N.J.: Lawrence Erlbaum.

Clement, J. (2004). "Imagistic processes in analogical reasoning: Conserving transformations and dual simulations." In *Proceedings of the Twenty-sixth Annual Conference of the Cognitive Science Society*. Mahwah, N.J.: Lawrence Erlbaum.

Clement, C. A., and D. Gentner (1991). "Systematicity as a selection constraint in analogical mapping." *Cognitive Science* 1: 89–132.

Clement, J. J., and M. S. Steinberg (2002). "Step-wise evolution of mental models of electric circuits: A 'learning-aloud' case study." *Journal of the Learning Sciences* 11 (4): 389–452.

Cooper, L. A., and R. N. Shepard (1973). "Chronometric studies of the rotation of mental images." In *Visual Information Processing*, 75–176, ed. W. G. Chase. New York: Academic Press.

Craig, D. L., N. J. Nersessian, and R. Catrambone (2002a). "Perceptual simulation in analogical problem solving." In *Model-Based Reasoning: Science, Technology, Values*, 167–190, ed. L. Magnani and N. J. Nersessian. New York: Kluwer Academic/ Plenum.

Craig, D. L., N. J. Nersessian, and R. Catrambone (2002b). "The role of diagrams and diagrammatic affordances in analogy." In *Proceedings of the Cognitive Science Society 24*, 250–255, ed. W. Gray and C. D. Schunn. Hillsdale, N.J.: Lawrence Erlbaum.

Craik, K. (1943). *The Nature of Explanation*. Cambridge: Cambridge University Press.

Croft, D., and P. Thagard (2002). "Dynamic imagery: A computational model of motion and visual analogy." In *Model-based Reasoning: Science, Technology, Values*, ed. L. Magnani and N. J. Nersessian. New York: Kluwer Academic/Plenum.

Crosbie Smith, M., and N. Wise (1989). *Energy and Empire: A Biographical Study of Lord Kelvin*. Cambridge: Cambridge University Press.

Darden, L. (1980). "Theory construction in genetics." In *Scientific Discovery: Case Studies* 60: 151–170, ed. T. Nickles. Dordrecht: Reidel.

Darden, L. (1991). *Theory Change in Science: Strategies from Mendelian Genetics*. New York: Oxford University Press.

Davies, G. E. (2000). *The Democratic Intellect*. Edinburgh: University of Edinburgh Press.

Davies, J. (2004). Constructive Adaptive Visual Analogy. College of Computing. Atlanta, Georgia Institute of Technology. Doctoral Dissertation.

Davies, D., N. J. Nersessian, and A. Goel (2005). "Visual models in analogical problem solving." *Foundations of Science* 10 (1): 133–152.

Dear, P. (1985). "Totius in verba: Rhetoric and Authority in the Early Royal Society." *Isis* 76: 145–161.

DeLoache, J. S. (1987). "Rapid change in the symbolic functioning of very young children." *Science* 238: 1556–1557.

Dennett, D. C. (2000). Making tools for thinking. *Metarepresentations: A Multidisciplinary Perspective*, 17–29, ed. D. Sperber. New York: Oxford University Press.

Dijk, T. A. V., and W. Kintsch (1983). *Strategies of Discourse Comprehension*. New York: Academic Press.

Donald, M. (1991). *Origins of the Modern Mind: Three Stages in the Evolution of Culture and Cognition*. Cambridge, Mass.: Harvard University Press.

Duhem, P. (1902). *Les théories électriques de J. Clerk Maxwell: Etude historique et critique*. Paris: A. Hermann & Cie.

Duhem, P. (1914). *The Aim and Structure of Physical Theory*. New York: Atheneum.

Dunbar, K. (1995). "How scientists really reason: Scientific reasoning in real-world laboratories." In *The Nature of Insight*, 365–395, ed. R. J. Sternberg and J. E. Davidson. Cambridge, Mass.: MIT Press.

Dunbar, K. (2000). "What scientific thinking reveals about the nature of cognition." In *Designing for Science: Implications for Everyday, Classroom, and Professional Settings*, 115–140, ed. K. Crowley, C. D. Schunn, and T. Okada. Hillsdale, N.J.: Lawrence Erlbaum.

Dunbar, K., and I. Blanchette (2001). "The *in vivo/in vitro* approach to cognition: The case of analogy." *Trends in Cognitive Science* 5: 334–339.

Duncker, K. O. (1945). "On problem solving." *Psychological Monographs* 58.

Duschl, R. A. (1990). *Restructuring Science Education: The Importance of Theories and Their Development*. New York: Teachers College Press.

Einstein, A. (1973). *Ideas and Opinions*. New York: Dell.

Einstein, A. (1985). Letter to Jacques Hadamard. In *The Creative Process: A Symposium*, ed. B. Ghiselin. Berkeley, Calif.: University of California Press.

Einstein, A. (1961). *Relativity: The Special and General Theory*. New York: Crown Publishers.

Elgin, C. Z. (1996). *Considered Judgment*. Princeton: Princeton University Press.

Elgin, C. Z. (2004). "True enough." *Philosophical Issues* 14: 113–131.

Elgin, C. Z. (in press). "Exemplification, idealization, and understanding." In *Fictions in Science: Essays on Idealization and Modeling*, ed. M. Suárez. London: Routledge,

Ericsson, K. A., and H. A. Simon (1984). *Protocol Analysis: Verbal Reports as Data*. Cambridge, Mass.: MIT Press.

Faraday, M. (183–1855). *Experimental Researches in Electricity*. 3 Volumes. New York: Dover.

Faraday, M. (1852a). "On Lines of Magnetic Force; Their Definite Character; and Their Distribution within a Magnet and through Space." *Philosophical Transactions* 142: 25–56.

Faraday, M. (1852). "On the Physical Character of the Lines of Magnetic Force." *Philosophical Magazine* 3: 401–428.

Faraday, M. (1932). *Diary*. Edited by T. Martin. 7 Volumes. London: G. Bell & Sons Ltd.

Farah, M. J. (1988). "Is visual imagery really visual? Overlooked evidence from neuropsychology." *Psychological Review* 95: 307–317.

Faries, J. M., and Reiser, B. J. (1988). "Access and use of previous solutions in a problem solving situation." In *Proceedings of the Tenth Annual Meeting of the Cognitive Science Society, Montreal*. Hillsdale, N.J.: Lawrence Erlbaum.

Feigl, H. (1970). "The 'orthodox' view of theories: Remarks in defense as well as critique." In *Analyses of Theories and Methods of Physics and Psychology* 4, ed. M. Radner and S. Winokur. Minneapolis: University of Minnesota Press.

Feist, G. J., and M. Gorman (1998). "The psychology of science." *Review of general psychology* 2: 3–47.

Ferguson, E. S. (1992). *Engineering and the Mind's Eye*. Cambridge, Mass.: MIT Press.

Ferguson, R. W. (1994). "MAGI: Analogy-based encoding using symmetry and regularity." In *Proceedings of the Sixteenth Cognitive Science Society Conference*. Hillsdale, N.J.: Lawrence Erlbaum.

Feyerabend, P. (1962). "Explanation, reduction, and empiricism." In *Minnesota Studies in the Philosophy of Science* 3, ed. H. Feigl and G. Maxwell. Pittsburgh: University of Pittsburgh Press.

Finke, R. A. (1989). *Principles of Mental Imagery*. Cambridge, Mass.: MIT Press.

Finke, R. A., S. Pinker, and M. Farah (1989). "Reinterpreting visual patterns in mental imagery." *Cognitive Science* 13: 51–78.

Finke, R. A., and R. N. Shepard (1986). "Visual functions of mental imagery." In *Handbook of Perception and Human Performance*, 37.1–37.55, ed. K. R. Boff et al. New York: Wiley.

Fodor, J. A. (1975). *The Language of Thought*. New York: Thomas Y. Crowell.

Forbus, K. (1983). "Reasoning about space and motion." In *Mental Models*, 53–74, ed. D. Gentner and A. Stevens. Hillsdale, N.J.: Lawrence Erlbaum.

Forbus, K., D. Gentner, and K. Law (1995). "MAC/FAC: A model of similarity-based retrieval." *Cognitive Science* 19 (2): 141–205.

Forbus, K. D., D. Gentner, A. B. Markman, and R. W. Ferguson (1998). "Analogy just looks like high-level perception: Why a domain-general approach to analogical mapping is right." *Journal of Experimental and Theoretical Artificial Intelligence* 10 (2): 231–257.

Franklin, N., and B. Tversky (1990). "Searching imagined environments." *Journal of Experimental Psychology* 119: 63–76.

French, R. (1995). *The Subtlety of Sameness: A Theory and Computer Model of Analogy-making* Cambridge, Mass.: MIT Press.

Freyd, J. J. (1987). "Dynamic mental representation." *Psychological Review* 94: 427–438.

Galantucci, B., C. A. Fowler, and Turvey, M. T. (2006). "The motor theory of speech perception reviewed." *Psychonomic Bulletin and Review* 13: 361–377.

Galilei, G. (1632/1967). *Dialogue Concerning Two Chief World Systems*. Berkeley, Calif.: University of California Press.

Galison, P. (1997). *Image and Logic: A Material Culture of Microphysics*. Chicago: University of Chicago Press.

Gallese, V., P. F. Ferrari, E. Kohler, and L. Fogassi (2002). "The eyes, the hand, and the mind: Behavioral and neurophysiological aspects of social cognition." In *The Cognitive Animal*, 451–462, ed. M. Bekoff, C. Allen, and M. Burghardt. Cambridge, Mass.: MIT Press.

Gatti, A. (2005). "On the nature of cognitive representations and on the cognitive role of manipulations: A case study: Surgery." In *Proceedings of the 26th Annual Conference of the Cognitive Science Society*. Hillsdale, N.J.: Lawrence Erlbaum.

Gattis, M., and K. J. Holyoak (1996). "Mapping conceptual to spatial relations in visual reasoning." *Journal of Experimental Psychology: Learning, Memory, and Cognition* 22: 231–239.

Geertz, C. (1973). *The Interpretation of Cultures*. New York: Basic Books.

Gentner, D. (1983). "Structure-mapping: A theoretical framework for analogy." *Cognitive Science* 7: 155–170.

Gentner, D., S. Brem, R. W. Ferguson, A. B. Markman, B. B. Levidow, P. Wolff, and K. D. Forbus (1997). "Analogical reasoning and conceptual change: A case study of Johannes Kepler." *Journal of the Learning Sciences* 6 (1): 3–40.

Gentner, D., and D. R. Gentner (1983). "Flowing waters and teeming crowds: Mental models of electricity." In *Mental Models*, 99–130, ed. D. Gentner and A. Stevens. Hillsdale, N.J.: Lawrence Erlbaum.

Gentner, D., and M. J. Ratterman (1991). "Language and the career of similarity." In *Perspective on Thought and Language: Interrelations in Development*, ed. S. Gelman and J. P. Byrnes. Cambridge: Cambridge University Press.

Gentner, D., M. J. Rattermann, and K. D. Forbus (1993). "The roles of similarity in transfer: Separating retrievability from inferential soundness." *Cognitive Psychology* 25: 524–575.

Gentner, D., and A. L. Stevens (1983). *Mental Models*. Hillsdale, N.J.: Lawrence Erlbaum.

Gentner, D., and C. Toupin (1986). "Systematicity and surface similarity in the development of analogy." *Cognitive Science* 10(3): 277–300.

Gibson, J. J. (1979). *The Ecological Approach to Visual Perception*. Boston: Houghton Mifflin.

Gick, M. L., and K. J. Holyoak (1980). "Analogical problem solving." *Cognitive Psychology* 12: 306–355.

Gick, M. L., and K. L. Holyoak (1983). "Schema induction and analogical transfer." *Cognitive Psychology* 15: 1–38.

Giere, R. N. (1988). *Explaining Science: A Cognitive Approach*. Chicago: University of Chicago Press.

Giere, R. N. (1992). *Cognitive Models of Science: Minnesota Studies in the Philosophy of Science 15*. Minneapolis: University of Minnesota Press.

Giere, R. N. (1994). "The cognitive structure of scientific theories." *Philosophy of Science* 61: 276–296.

Gilbert, J. K., and C. J. Boulter (2000). *Developing Models in Science Education*. Dordrecht: Kluwer Academic.

Gilhooly, K. J. (1986). "Mental modeling: A framework for the study of thinking." In *Thinking: Progress in Research and Teaching*, 19–32, ed. J. Bishop, J. Lochhead, and D. Perkins. Hillsdale, N.J.: Lawrence Erlbaum.

Glasgow, J. I., N. H. Narayanan, and B. Chandrasekaran (eds.) (1995). *Diagrammatic Reasoning: Cognitive and Computational Perspectives*, Menlo Park, Calif.: AAAI Press.

Glenberg, A. M. (1997a). "What memory is for." *Behavioral and Brain Sciences* 20: 1–55.

Glenberg, A. M. (1997b). "Mental models, space, and embodied cognition." In *Creative Thought: An Investigation of Conceptual Structures and Processes*, 495–522, ed. T. Ward, S. M. Smith, and J. Vaid. Washington, D.C.: American Psychological Association.

Glenberg, A. M., and W. E. Langston (1992). "Comprehension of illustrated text: Pictures help to build mental models." *Journal of Memory and Language* 31: 129–151.

Gobert, J., and B. Buckley (2000). "Special issue editorial: Introduction to model-based teaching and learning." *International Journal of Science Education* 22 (9): 891–894.

Gobert, J., and J. Clement (1999). " Effects of student-generated diagrams versus student-generated summaries on conceptual understanding of causal and dynamic knowledge in plate tectonics." *Journal of Research in Science Teaching* 36 (1): 39–53.

Godfrey-Smith, P. (2006). "The Strategy of Model-Based Science." *Biology and Philosophy* 21: 721–40.

Goldin-Meadow, S., H. Nusbaum, S. D. Kelly, and S. Wagner (2001). "Explaining math: Gesturing lightens the load." *Psychological Science* 12 (6): 332–340.

Goldin-Meadow, S., and S. M. Wagner (2005). "How our hands help us learn." *Trends in Cognitive Science* 9: 234–240.

Goldman, A. I. (1986). *Epistemology and Cognition*. Cambridge, Mass.: Harvard University Press.

Gooding, D. (1980). "Faraday, Thomson, and the concept of magnetic field." *British Journal for the History of Science* 13: 91–120.

Gooding, D. (1981). "Final steps to the field theory: Faraday's study of electromagnetic phenomena, 1845–1850." *Historical Studies in the Physical Sciences* 11: 231–275.

Gooding, D. (1990). *Experiment and the Making of Meaning: Human Agency in Scientific Observation and Experiment*. Dordrecht: Kluwer.

Gooding, D. C. (2004). "Cognition, construction, and culture: Visual theories in the sciences." *Journal of Cognition and Culture* 4 (3–4): 551–593.

Gooding, D. (2005). "Seeing the forest for the trees: Visualization, cognition, and scientific inference." In *Scientific and Technological Thinking*, 173–218, ed. M. Gorman, R. D. Tweney, D. Gooding, and A. Kincannon. Mahwah, N.J.: Lawrence Erlbaum.

Goodman, N. (1968). *Languages of Art*. Indianapolis: Hackett.

Gorman, M. (1997). "Mind in the world: Cognition and practice in the invention of the telephone." *Social Studies of Science* 27: 583–624.

Goswami, U. (1992). *Analogical Reasoning in Children*. East Sussex: Lawrence Erlbaum.

Goswami, U., and A. L. Brown (1989). "Melting chocolate and melting snowmen: Analogical reasoning and causal relations." *Cognition* 35: 69–95.

Greeno, J. G. (1989). "Situations, mental models, and generative knowledge." In *Complex Information Processing*, 285–318, ed. D. Klahr and K. Kotovsky. Hillsdale, N.J.: Lawrence Erlbaum.

Greeno, J. G. (1998). "The situativity of knowing, learning, and research. *American Psychologist* 53: 5–24.

Griesemer, J. R. (1991a). "Must scientific diagrams be eliminable? The case of path analysis." *Biology and Philosophy* 6: 177–202.

Griesemer, J. R. (1991b). "Material models in biology." *PSA* 2: 79–94.

Griesemer, J. R., and W. Wimsatt (1989). "Picturing Weismannism: A case study of conceptual evolution." In *What the Philosophy of Biology Is: Essays for David Hull*, 75–137, ed. M. Ruse. Dordrecht: Kluwer.

Griffith, T. W. (1999). "A Computational Theory of Generative Modeling in Scientific Reasoning." College of Computing. Atlanta, Georgia Institute of Technology. Doctoral dissertation.

Griggs, R. A., and J. R. Cox (1993). "Permission schemas and the selection task." *Quarterly Journal of Experimental Psychology* 46A: 637–651.

Hanson, N. R. (1958). *Patterns of Discovery*. Cambridge: Cambridge University Press.

Harman [Heimann], P. M. (1990). *The Scientific Papers and Letters of James Clerk Maxwell*, volume 1. Cambridge: Cambridge University Press.

Harman [Heimann], P. M. (1995). *The Scientific Letters and Papers of James Clerk Maxwell*, volume 2. Cambridge: Cambridge University Press.

Harnad, S. (1990). "The symbol grounding problem." *Physica D* 42: 35–46.

Haugeland, J. (1991). "Representational genera." In *Philosophy and Connectionist Theory*, ed. W. Ramsey, S. Stitch, and D. E. Rumelhart. Hillsdale, N.J.: Lawrence Erlbaum.

Hayes, P. J. (1979). "The naive physics manifesto." In *Expert Systems in the Micro-Electronic Age*, ed. D. Mitchie. Edinburgh: Edinburgh University Press.

Hegarty, M. (1992). "Mental animation: Inferring motion from static diagrams of mechanical systems." *Journal of Experimental Psychology: Learning, Memory, and Cognition* 18 (5): 1084–1102.

Hegarty, M. (2004). "Diagrams in the mind and in the world: Relations between internal and external visualizations." In *Diagrammatic Representation and Inference*, ed. A. Blackwell, K. Mariott, and A. Shimojima. Berlin: Springer.

Hegarty, M. (2004). "Mechanical reasoning by mental simulation." *Trends in Cognitive Science* 8: 280–285.

Hegarty, M., and J. M. Ferguson (1993). "Strategy change with practice in a mental animation task." Paper presented at the Annual Meeting of the Psychonomic Society, Washington, D.C.

Hegarty, M., and M. A. Just (1989). "Understanding machines from text and diagrams." In *Knowledge Acquisition from Text and Picture*, ed. H. Mandl and J. Levin. Amsterdam: North Holland, Elsevier Science Publishers.

Hegarty, M., and V. K. Sims (1994). "Individual differences in mental animation from text and diagrams." *Journal of Memory and Language* 32: 411–430.

Hegarty, M., and K. Steinhoff (1997). "Use of diagrams as external memory in a mechanical reasoning task." *Learning and Individual Differences* 9: 19–42.

Heimann, P. M. (1970). "Maxwell and the modes of consistent representation." *Archive for the History of Exact Sciences* 6: 171–213.

Hempel, C. G. (1952). *Fundamentals of Concept Formation in Empirical Science*. Chicago: University of Chicago Press.

Hesse, M. (1963). *Models and Analogies in Science*. London: Sheed and Ward.

Hesse, M. (1973). "Logic of discovery in Maxwell's electromagnetic theory." In *Foundations of Scientific Method: The 19th Century*, 86–114, ed. R. N. Giere and R. S. Westfall. Bloomington: University of Indiana Press.

Hoffman, J. R. (1996). *Andre-Marie Ampere*. Cambridge: Cambridge University Press.

Hofstadter, D. (1995). *Fluid Concepts and Creative Analogies: Computer Models of the Fundamental Mechanisms of Thought*. New York: Basic Books.

Holland, J. H., K. J. Holyoak, R. E. Nisbett, and P. R. Thagard (1986). *Induction: Processes of Inference, Learning, and Discovery*. Cambridge, Mass.: MIT Press.

Holmes, F. L. (1981). "The fine structure of scientific creativity." *History of Science* 19: 60–70.

Holmes, F. L. (1985). *Lavoisier and the Chemistry of Life: An Exploration of Scientific Creativity*. Madison: University of Wisconsin Press.

Holmes, F. L. (1990). "Argument and narrative in scientific writing." In *The Paper Laboratory: Textual Strategies, Literary Genres, and Disciplinary Traditions in the History of Science*, 164–181, ed. P. Dear. Philadelphia: University of Pennsylvania Press.

Holyoak, K. J., E. N. Junn, and D. Billman (1984). "Development of analogical problem-solving skill." *Child Development* 55: 2042–2055.

Holyoak, K. J., and P. Thagard (1996). *Mental Leaps: Analogy in Creative Thought.* Cambridge, Mass.: MIT Press.

Hurley, S., and N. Chater (eds.) (2005a). *Imitation, Human Development, and Culture.* Perspectives on Imitation: From Neuroscience to Social Science. Cambridge, Mass.: MIT Press.

Hurley, S., and N. Chater (eds.) (2005b). *Mechanisms of Imitation in Animals.* Perspectives on Imitation: From Neuroscience to Social Science. Cambridge, Mass.: MIT Press.

Hutchins, E. (1995a). *Cognition in the Wild.* Cambridge, Mass.: MIT Press.

Hutchins, E. (1995b). "How a cockpit remembers its speed." *Cognitive Science* 19: 265–288.

Inhelder, B., and Piaget, J. (1958). *The Growth of Logical Thinking from Childhood to Adolescence: An Essay on the Construction of Formal Operational Structures.* New York: Basic Books.

Jackson, J. D. (1962). *Classical Electrodynamics.* New York: John Wiley.

Jeannerod, M. (1993). "A theory of representation-driven actions." In *The Perceived Self*, 68–88, ed. U. Neisser. Cambridge: Cambridge University Press.

Jeannerod, M. (1994). "The representing brain: Neural correlated of motor intention and imagery." *Brain and Behavioral Sciences* 17: 187–202.

Johnson, M. (1987). *The Body in the Mind: The Bodily Basis of Meaning, Imagination, and Reason.* Chicago: University of Chicago Press.

Johnson-Laird, P. N. (1980). "Mental models in cognitive science." *Cognitive Science* 4: 71–115.

Johnson-Laird, P. N. (1982). "The mental representation of the meaning of words." *Cognition* 25: 189–211.

Johnson-Laird, P. N. (1983). *Mental Models.* Cambridge, Mass.: MIT Press.

Johnson-Laird, P. N. (1984). "Deductive thinking: How we reason." In *Handbook of Cognitive Neuroscience.* New York: Plenum.

Johnson-Laird, P. N. (1989). "Mental models." In *Foundations of Cognitive Science*, 469–500, ed. M. Posner. Cambridge, Mass.: MIT Press.

Johnson-Laird, P. N. (1990). "Human thinking and mental models." In *Modelling the Mind*, ed. K. A. Mohyeldin Said, W. H. Newton-Smith, R. Viale, and K. V. Wilkes. Oxford: Clarendon Press.

Johnson-Laird, P. M. (1995). "Models in deductive thinking." In *The Cognitive Neurosciences*, 999–1008, ed. M. S. Gazzaniga. Cambridge, Mass.: MIT Press.

Johnson-Laird, P. N. (2002). "Peirce, logic diagrams, and the elementary operations of reasoning." *Thinking and Reasoning* 8: 69–95.

Johnson-Laird, P. N., and R. Byrne (1991). *Deduction*. Hove: Lawrence Erlbaum.

Johnson-Laird, P. N., and R. Byrne (1993). "Precis of the book *Deduction* with peer review commentaries and responses." *Brain and Behavioral Sciences* 16: 323–380.

Johnson-Laird, P. N., P. Legrenzi, and M. Sonino Legrenzi (1972). "Reasoning and a sense of reality." *British Journal of Psychology* 63: 395–400.

Justi, R., and J. Gilbert (1999). "A cause of ahistorical science teaching: Use of hybrid models." *Science Education* 83: 163–177.

Kahneman, D., and A. Tversky (1982). *Judgement under Uncertainty: Heuristics and Biases*. New York: Cambridge University Press.

Keane, M. (1985). "On drawing analogies when solving problems: A theory and test of solution generation in analogical problem-solving tasks." *British Journal of Psychology* 76: 449–458.

Kempton, W. (1986). "Two theories of home heat control." *Cognitive Science* 10: 75–90.

Kerr, N. H. (1983). "The role of vision in 'visual imagery.'" *Journal of Experimental Psychology: General* 112: 265–277.

Kirsh, D. (1995). "Complementary strategies: Why we use our hands when we think." In *Proceedings of the Seventeenth Annual Conference of the Cognitive Science Society*. Hillsdale, N.J.: Lawrence Erlbaum.

Kirsh, D., and P. Maglio (1994). "On distinguishing epistemic from pragmatic action." *Cognitive Science* 18: 513–549.

Kitcher, P. (1993). *The Advancement of Science*. New York: Oxford University Press.

Klahr, D., and H. A. Simon (1999). "Studies of scientific discovery: Complementary approaches and divergent findings." *Psychological Bulletin* 125: 524–543.

Koedinger, K., and J. R. Anderson (1990). "Abstract planning and perceptual chunks: Elements of expertise in geometry." *Cognitive Science* 14: 511–550.

Koestler, A. (1964). *The Act of Creation*. London: Penguin Books.

Kolodner, J. L. (1993). *Case-based Reasoning*. San Mateo, Calif. Morgan Kaufmann.

Kosslyn, S. M. (1980). *Image and Mind*. Cambridge, Mass.: Harvard University Press.

Kosslyn, S. M. (1994). *Image and Brain*. Cambridge, Mass.: MIT Press.

Kuhn, T. (1962). *The Structure of Scientific Revolutions: International Encyclopedia of Unified Science*. Chicago: University of Chicago Press.

Kuhn, T. (1970). *The Structure of Scientific Revolutions*. Chicago: University of Chicago Press.

Kuhn, T. S. (1977). *The Essential Tension: Selected Studies in Scientific Tradition and Change*. Chicago: University of Chicago Press.

Kurz, E. M., and R. D. Tweney (1998). "The practice of mathematics and science: From calculus to the clothesline problem." In *Rational Models of Cognition*, 415–438, ed. M. Oakfield and N. Chater. London: Oxford University Press.

Lakoff, G. (1987). *Women, Fire, and Dangerous Things: What Categories Reveal about the Mind*. Chicago: University of Chicago Press.

Lakoff, G., and M. Johnson (1998). *Philosophy in the Flesh*. New York: Basic Books.

Larkin, J. H. (1989). "Display-based problem solving." In *Complex Information Processing: The Impact of Herbert A. Simon*, 319–342, ed. D. Klahr and K. Kotovsky. Hillsdale, N.J.: Lawrence Erlbaum.

Larkin, J. H., and H. A. Simon (1987). "Why a diagram is (sometimes) worth ten thousand words." *Cognitive Science* 11: 65–100.

Larmor, J. (ed.) (1937). *The Origins of Clerk Maxwell's Electric Ideas*. Cambridge: Cambridge University Press.

Laudan, L. (1977). *Progress and Its Problems: Towards a Theory of Scientific Growth*. Cambridge, Mass.: MIT Press.

Lave, J. (1988). *Cognition in Practice: Mind, Mathematics, and Culture in Everyday Life*. New York: Cambridge University Press.

Longino, H. (2001). *The Fate of Knowledge*. Princeton: Princeton University Press.

Magnani, L., N. J. Nersessian, and P. Thagard (eds.) (1999). *Model-Based Reasoning in Scientific Discovery*. New York; Kluwer Academic/Plenum.

Mainwaring, S. D., B. Tversky, and D. Schiano (1996). "Effects of task and object configuration on perspective choice in spatial descriptions." In *AAAI Symposium*, 56–67, ed. P. Olivier. Stanford, Calif.: AAAI Press.

Mani, K., and P. N. Johnson-Laird (1982). "The mental representation of spatial descriptions." *Memory and Cognition* 10: 181–187.

Marmor, G. S., and L. A. Zaback (1976). "Mental rotation by the blind: Does mental rotation depend on visual imagery?" *Journal of Experimental Psychology: Human Perception and Performance* 2: 515–521.

Maxwell, J. C. (1855–1856). "On Faraday's lines of force." *Scientific Papers* 1: 155–229, ed. W. D. Niven. Cambridge: Cambridge University Press.

Maxwell, J. C. (1856). "Are there real analogies in nature?" In *The Life of James Clerk Maxwell*, 235–244, ed. L. Campbell and W. Garnett. London, Macmillan.

Maxwell, J. C. (1861–1862). "On physical lines of force." In *Scientific Papers* 1, 451–513, ed. W. D. Niven. Cambridge: Cambridge University Press.

Maxwell, J. C. (1864). "A dynamical theory of the electromagnetic field." In *Scientific Papers* 1, 526–597, ed. W. D. Niven. Cambridge: Cambridge University Press.

Maxwell, J. C. (1873). "Quaternions." *Nature* 9 (217): 137–138.

Maxwell, J. C. (1876). "On the Proof of the Equations of Motion of a Connected System." In *Scientific Papers* 2, 308–309, ed. W. D. Niven. Cambridge: Cambridge University Press.

Maxwell, J. C. (1890a). *The Scientific Papers of James Clerk Maxwell*, ed. W. D. Niven. 2 volumes. Cambridge: Cambridge University.

Maxwell, J. C. (1890b). "On the mathematical classification of physical quantities." In *Scientific Papers* 2, 257–266, ed. W. D. Niven. Cambridge: Cambridge University.

Maxwell, J. C. (1891). *A Treatise on Electricity and Magnetism*, 3rd edition. Oxford: Clarendon.

McNamara, T. P., and R. J. Sternberg (1983). "Mental models of word meaning." *Journal of Verbal Learning and Verbal Behavior* 22: 449–474.

Metzinger, T. G., and V. Gallese (2003). "The emergence of a shared action ontology: Building blocks for a theory." *Consciousness and Cognition* 12 (Special Issue on Grounding the Self in Action): 549–571.

Miščević, N. (1992). "Mental models and thought experiments." *International Studies in the Philosophy of Science* 6: 215–226.

Mitchell, M. (1993). *Analogy-making as Perception: A Computer Model*. Cambridge, Mass.: MIT Press.

Morgan, M. S., and M. Morrison (eds.) (1999). *Models as Mediators*. Cambridge: Cambridge University Press.

Morrow, D. G., G. H. Bower, and S. L. Greenspan (1989). "Updating situation models during narrative comprehension." *Journal of Memory and Language* 28: 292–312.

Nersessian, N. J. (1984a). *Faraday to Einstein: Constructing Meaning in Scientific Theories*. Dordrecht: Martinus Nijhoff/Kluwer Academic.

Nersessian, N. J. (1984b). "Aether/or: The creation of scientific concepts." *Studies in the History and Philosophy of Science* 15: 175–212.

Nersessian, N. J. (1985). "Faraday's field concept." In *Faraday Rediscovered: Essays on the Life and Work of Michael Faraday*, 377–406, ed. D. C. Gooding and F. A. J. L. James. London: Macmillan.

Nersessian, N. J. (1987). "A cognitive-historical approach to meaning in scientific theories." In *The Process of Science*, 161–179. Dordrecht: Kluwer Academic.

Nersessian, N. J. (1989). "Conceptual change in science and in science education." *Synthese* 80 (Special Issue: Philosophy of Science and Science Education): 163–184.

Nersessian, N. J. (1991). "Why do thought experiments work?" In *Proceedings of the Cognitive Science Society 13*, 430–438. Hillsdale, N.J.: Lawrence Erlbaum.

Nersessian, N. J. (1992a). "How do scientists think? Capturing the dynamics of conceptual change in science." In *Minnesota Studies in the Philosophy of Science*, 3–45, ed. R. Giere. Minneapolis: University of Minnesota Press.

Nersessian, N. J. (1992b). "In the theoretician's laboratory: Thought experimenting as mental modeling." In *PSA 1992*, 2: 291–301, ed. D. Hull, M. Forbes, and K. Okruhlik. East Lansing, Mich.: PSA.

Nersessian, N. J. (1992c). "Constructing and Instructing: The Role of 'Abstraction Techniques' in Developing and Teaching Scientific Theories." In *Philosophy of Science, Cognitive Science, and Educational Theory and Practice*, 48–68, eds. R. Duschl and R. Hamilton. Albany, N.Y.: SUNY Press.

Nersessian, N. J. (1995a). "Opening the black box: Cognitive science and the history of science." *Osiris* 10 (Constructing Knowledge in the History of Science, ed. A. Thackray): 194–211.

Nersessian, N. J. (1995b). "Should Physicists Preach What They Practice? Constructive Modeling in Doing and Learning Physics." *Science and Education* 4: 203–226.

Nersessian, N. J. (2001). "Conceptual change and commensurability." In *Incommensurability and Related Matters*, 275–301, ed. H. Sankey and P. Hoyningen-Huene. Dordrecht: Kluwer Academic.

Nersessian, N. J. (2002a). "Kuhn, conceptual change, and cognitive science." In *Thomas Kuhn*, 178–211, ed. T. Nickles. Cambridge: Cambridge University Press.

Nersessian, N. J. (2002b). "The cognitive basis of model-based reasoning in science." In *The Cognitive Basis of Science*, 133–153, ed. P. Carruthers, S. Stich, and M. Siegal. Cambridge: Cambridge University Press.

Nersessian, N. J. (2002c). "Maxwell and the 'method of physical analogy': Model-based reasoning, generic abstraction, and conceptual change." In *Reading Natural Philosophy: Essays in the History and Philosophy of Science and Mathematics*, 129–165, ed. D. Malament. Lasalle, Ill.: Open Court.

Nersessian, N. J. (2003). "Abstraction via generic modeling in concept formation in science." *Mind and Society* 3: 129–154.

Nersessian, N. J. (2005). "Interpreting scientific and engineering practices: Integrating the cognitive, social, and cultural dimensions." In *Scientific and Technological Thinking*, 17–56, ed. M. Gorman, R. D. Tweney, D. Gooding, and A. Kincannon. Hillsdale, N.J.: Lawrence Erlbaum.

Nersessian, N. J. (2006). "The cognitive-cultural systems of the research laboratory." *Organization Studies* 27: 125–145.

Nersessian, N. J. (2008). "Mental modeling in conceptual change." In *International Handbook of Conceptual Change*, ed. S. Vosniadou. London: Routledge.

Nersessian, N. J., and H. Andersen (1997). "Conceptual Change and Incommensurability: A Cognitive-Historical View." *Danish Yearbook of Philosophy* 32: 111–151.

Nersessian, N. J., E. Kurz-Milcke, W. Newstetter, and J. Davies (2003). "Research laboratories as evolving distributed cognitive systems." In *Proceedings of the Cognitive Science Society 25*, 857–862, ed. D. Alterman and D. Kirsch. Hillsdale, N.J.: Lawrence Erlbaum.

Nersessian, N. J., and C. Patton (in press). "Model-based reasoning in interdisciplinary engineering: Two case studies from biomedical engineering research laboratories." In *Philosophy of Technology and Engineering Sciences*, ed. A. Meijers. Amsterdam: Elsevier Science.

Nisbett, R., K. Peng, I. Choi, and A. Norenzayan (2001). "Culture and systems of thought: Holistic v. analytic cognition." *Psychological Review* 108 (2): 291–310.

Norman, D. A. (1981). *Perspectives on Cognitive Science*. Hillsdale, N.J.: Lawrence Erlbaum.

Norman, D. A. (1988). *The Psychology of Everyday Things*. New York: Basic Books.

Norman, D. A. (1991). "Cognitive artifacts." In *Designing Interaction*, ed. J. M. Carroll. Cambridge: Cambridge University Press.

Norton, J. (1991). "Thought experiments in Einstein's work." In *Thought Experiments in Science and Philosophy*, 129–148, ed. T. Horowitz and G. Massey. Savage, Maryland: Rowman and Littlefield.

Norton, J. (2004). "Why thought experiments do not transcend empiricism." In *Contemporary Debates in the Philosophy of Science*, 44–66, ed. C. Hitchcock. Oxford, Blackwell.

Novick, L. (1988). "Analogical transfer, problem similarity, and expertise." *Journal of Experimental Psychology: Learning, Memory, and Cognition* 14 (3): 510–520.

Osbeck, L., and N. J. Nersessian (2006). "The distribution of representation." *Journal for the Theory of Social Behaviour* 36: 141–160.

Parsons, L. (1987). "Imagined spatial transformation of one's body." *Journal of Experimental Psychology: General* 116: 172–191.

Parsons, L. (1994). "Temporal and kinematic properties of motor behavior reflected in mentally simulated action." *Journal of Experimental Psychology: Human Perception and Performance* 20: 709–730.

Pedone, R., J. E. Hummell, and K. J. Holyoak (2001). "The use of diagrams in analogical problem solving." *Memory and Cognition* 29: 214–221.

Perrig, W., and W. Kintsch (1985). "Propositional and situational representations of text." *Journal of Memory and Language* 24: 503–518.

Peirce, C. S. (1931–1935). *Collected Papers of Charles Sanders Peirce*, volumes I–VI, ed. Charles Hartshorne and Paul Weiss. Cambridge, Mass.: Harvard University Press.

Polya, G. (1954). *Induction and Analogy in Mathematics*. Princeton: Princeton University Press.

Premack, D. (1983). "The codes of man and beast." *Behavioral and Brain Sciences* 6: 125–167.

Prinz, J. J. (2002). *Furnishing the Mind: Concepts and Their Perceptual Basis*. Cambridge, Mass.: MIT Press.

Prinz, W. (2005). "An ideomotor approach to imitation." In *Perspectives on Imitation: From Neuroscience to Social Science*, volume 1, 141–156, ed. S. Hurley and N. Chater. Cambridge, Mass.: MIT Press.

Quine, W. V. O. (1951). Two dogmas of empiricism. *Philosophical Review* 60: 20–43. Reprinted in W. V. O. Quine, *From a Logical Point of View* (Cambridge, Mass.: Harvard University Press, 1953).

Quine, W. V. O. (1970). "Epistemology Naturalized." In *Ontological Relativity and Other Essays*, 69–90. New York: Columbia University Press.

Reed, E. S. (1996). *Encountering the World: Toward an Ecological Psychology*. Oxford: Oxford University Press.

Reiner, M. (2004). "The role of haptics in immersive telecommunications environments." *IEEE Transactions on Circuits and Systems for Video Technology* 14 (3): 392–401.

Resnick, L. B., J. Levine, and S. Teasley (eds.) (1991). *Perspectives on Socially Shared Cognition*. Washington, D.C.: APA Press.

Rips, L. (1986). "Mental muddles." In *The Representation of Knowledge and Belief*, 258–286, ed. H. Brand and R. Hernish. Tucson: University of Arizona Press.

Rock, I. (1973). *Orientation and Form*. New York: Academic Press.

Ross, B. H. (1989). "Distinguishing types of superficial similarities: Different effects on the access and use of earlier examples." *Journal of Experimental Psychology: Learning, Memory, and Cognition* 15: 456–468.

Rouse, W. B., and N. M. Morris (1986). "On looking into the black box: Prospects and limits in the search for mental models." *Psychological Bulletin* 100 (3): 349–363.

Rudwick, M. J. S. (1976). "The emergence of a visual language for geological science." *History of Science* 14: 149–195.

Russell, B. (1924). "Logical atomism." In *Contemporary British Philosophy: Personal Statements (First series)*, ed. J. H. Muirhead. Library of Philosophy. London: Allen and Unwin.

Scaife, M., and Y. Rogers (1996). "External cognition: How do graphical representations work?" *International Journal of Human-Computer Studies* 45: 185–213.

Schumacher, R. M., and D. Gentner (1988). "Transfer of training as analogical mapping." *IEEE Transactions of Systems, Man, and Cybernetics* 18: 592–600.

Schwartz, D. L. (1995). "Reasoning about the referent of a picture versus reasoning about a the picture as the referent." *Memory and Cognition* 23: 709–722.

Schwartz, D. L., and J. B. Black (1996a). "Shuttling between depictive models and abstract rules: Induction and fall back." *Cognitive Science* 20: 457–497.

Schwartz, D. L., and J. B. Black (1996b). "Analog imagery in mental model reasoning: Depictive models." *Cognitive Psychology* 30: 154–219.

Searle, J. (1980). "Minds, brains, and programs." *Behavioral and Brain Sciences* 3: 417–424.

Sellars, W. (1973). "Givenness and explanatory coherence." *Journal of Philosophy* 70: 612–620.

Shapere, D. (1982). "The concept of observation in science and philosophy." *Philosophy of Science* 49: 485–525.

Shapin, S. (1984). "Pump and circumstance: Robert Boyle's literary technology." *Social Studies of Science* 14: 481–520.

Shelley, C. (1996). "Visual abductive reasoning in archeology." *Philosophy of Science* 63: 278–301.

Shepard, R. N. (1984). "Ecological constraints on internal representation: Resonant kinematics of perceiving, imagining, thinking, and dreaming." *Psychological Review* 91: 417–447.

Shepard, R. (1988). "Imagination of the scientist." In *Imagination and the Scientist*, 153–185, ed. K. Egan and D. Nadaner. New York: Teachers College Press.

Shepard, R. N. (1994). "Perceptual-cognitive universals as reflections of the world." *Psychonomic Bulletin and Review* 1: 2–28.

Shepard, R. N., and L. A. Cooper (1982). *Mental Images and Their Transformations*. Cambridge, Mass.: MIT Press.

Shiffrar, M., and J. J. Freyd (1990). "Apparent motion of the human body." *Psychological Science* 1: 257–264.

Shimojima, A. (2001). "The graphic-linguistic distinction." In *Thinking with Diagrams*, 5–28, ed. A. F. Blackwell. Dordrecht: Kluwer Academic.

Shore, B. (1997). *Culture in Mind: Cognition, Culture, and the Problem of Meaning*. New York: Oxford University Press.

Siegel, D. (1986). "The origin of the displacement current." *Historical Studies in the Physical Sciences* 17: 99–145.

Siegel, D. (1991). *Innovation in Maxwell's Electromagnetic Theory*. Cambridge: Cambridge University Press.

Simmons, W. K., S. B. Hamann, C. L. Nolan, X. Hu, and L. W. Barsalou (2004). "fMRI evidence for the role of word association and situation simulation in conceptual processing." Paper presented at the Meeting of the Society for Cognitive Neuroscience, San Francisco.

Simon, H. A. (1977). *Models of Thought*. Dordrecht: D. Reidel.

Smith, C., D. Maclin, L. Grosslight, and H. Davis (1997). "Teaching for understanding: A study of students' pre-instruction theories of matter and a comparison of the effectiveness of two approaches to teaching about matter and density." *Cognition and Instruction* 15 (3): 317–393.

Smith, C., J. Snir, and L. Grosslight (1992). "Using conceptual models to facilitate conceptual change: The case of weight-density differentiation." *Cognition and Instruction* 9 (3): 221–283.

Snir, J., and C. Smith (1995). "Constructing understanding in the science classroom: Integrating laboratory experiments, student and computer models, and class discussion in learning scientific concepts." In *Software Goes to School*, 233–254, ed. D. Perkins, J. Schwartz, M. West, and S. Wiske. Oxford: Oxford University Press.

Solomon, K. O., and L. W. Barsalou (2004). "Perceptual simulation in property verification." *Memory and Cognition* 32: 244–259.

Spelke, E. S. (1991). "Physical knowledge in infancy: Reflections on Piaget's theory." In *The Epigenesis of Mind: Essays on Biology and Cognition*, 133–169, ed. S. Carey and R. Gelman. Hillsdale, N.J.: Lawrence Erlbaum.

Spelke, E. S., A. Phillips, and A. L. Woodward (1995). "Spatio-temporal continuity, smoothness of motion and object identity in infancy." *British Journal of Developmental Psychology* 13: 113–142.

Spranzi, M. (2004). "Galileo and the mountains of the moon: Analogical reasoning, models and metaphors in scientific discovery." *Cognition and Culture* 4 (3): 4451–4485.

Star, S. L., and J. G. Griesemer (1989). "Institutional ecology, 'translations,' and boundary objects: Amateurs and professionals in Berkeley's Museum of Vertebrate Zoology, 1907–39." *Social Studies of Science* 19: 387–420.

Stein, H. (1976). "On action at a distance: Metaphysics and method in Newton and Maxwell." Unpublished talk, Yale University.

Steiner, M. (1989). "The application of mathematics to natural science." *Journal of Philosophy* 86 (9): 449–480.

Stenning, K. (2002). *Seeing Reason: Image and Language in Learning to Think*. London: Oxford University Press.

Stenning, K., and O. Lemon (2001). "Aligning logical and psychological perspectives on diagrammatic reasoning." *Artificial Intelligence Review* 15 (1/2): 29–62.

Stenning, K., and J. Oberlander (1995). "A theory of graphical and linguistic reasoning." *Cognitive Science* 19: 97–140.

Suarez, M. (2003). "Scientific representation: Against similarity and isomorphism." *International Studies in the Philosophy of Science* 17 (3): 225–244.

Suchman, L. A. (1987). *Plans and Situated Actions: The Problem of Human-Machine Communication*. Cambridge and New York: Cambridge University Press.

Svenson, H., and T. Ziemke (2004). *Making Sense of Embodiment: Simulation Theories and the Sharing of Neural Circuitry between Sensorimotor and Cognitive Processes*. Proceedings of the 26th Annual Meeting of the Cognitive Science Society, Chicago. Hillsdale, N.J.: Lawrence Erlbaum.

Tabachneck-Schijf, H. J. M., A. M. Leonardo, and H. A. Simon (1997). "CaMeRa: A computational model of multiple representations." *Cognitive Science* 21 (3): 305–350.

Thagard, P. (1988). *Computational Philosophy of Science*. Cambridge, Mass.: MIT Press.

Thagard, P. (1992). *Conceptual Revolutions*. Princeton: Princeton University Press.

Thagard, P., D. Gochfield, and S. Hardy (1992). "Visual analogical mapping." In *Fourteenth Annual Conference of the Cognitive Science Society*. Hillsdale, N.J.: Lawrence Erlbaum.

Thomson, W. (1845). "On the elementary laws of statical electricity." In *Reprint of Papers on Electrostatics and Magnetism*, 2nd edition, 14–37 (London: Macmillan, 1884).

Thomson, W. (1847). "On a mechanical representation of electric, magnetic, and galvanic forces." In *Mathematical and Physical Papers* I, 76–80. Cambridge: Cambridge University Press.

Thomson, W. (1851). "On the dynamical theory of heat, with numerical results deduced from Mr. Joule's equivalent of a thermal unit, and M. Regnault's observations on steam." In *Mathematical and Physical Papers* I, 174–232. Cambridge: Cambridge University Press.

Thomson, W. (1856) "Dynamical illustrations of the magnetic and heliocoidal rotatory effects of transparent bodies on polarized light." *Proceedings of the Royal Society* 8: 150–158.

Tomasello, M. (1999). *The Cultural Origins of Human Cognition*. Cambridge, Mass.: Harvard University Press.

Trafton, J. G., S. B. Trickett, and F. E. Mintz (2005). "Connecting internal and external representations: Spatial transformations of scientific visualizations." *Foundations of Science* 10: 89–106.

Trumpler, M. (1997). "Converging images: Techniques of intervention and forms of representation of sodium-channel proteins in nerve cell membranes." *Journal of the History of Biology* 20: 55–89.

Tversky, B., J. Zacks, P. U. Lee, and J. Heiser (2000). "Lines, blobs, crosses, and arrows: Diagrammatic communication with schematic figures." In *Theory and Application of Diagrams*, 221–230, ed. M. Andersen, P. Chang, and V. Haarslev. Berlin: Springer.

Tweney, R. D. (1985). "Faraday's discovery of induction: A cognitive approach." In *Faraday Rediscovered*, 189–210, ed. D. Gooding and F. A. J. L. James. New York: Stockton Press.

Tweney, R. D. (1987). "What is scientific thinking?" Unpublished manuscript.

Tweney, R. D. (1989). "Fields of enterprise: On Michael Faraday's thought." In *Creative People at Work*, 91–106, ed. D. B. Wallace and H. E. Gruber. New York: Oxford University Press.

Tweney, R. D. (1992). "Stopping time: Faraday and the scientific creation of perceptual order." *Physics* 29: 149–164.

Tye, M. (1991). *The Imagery Debate*. Cambridge, Mass.: MIT Press.

Vera, A., and H. Simon (1993). "Situated cognition: A symbolic interpretation." *Cognitive Science* 17: 4–48.

Vosniadou, S., and W. F. Brewer (1992). "Mental models of the earth: A study of conceptual change in childhood." *Cognitive Psychology* 24: 535–585.

Vygotsky, L. (1962). *Thought and Language*. Trans. E. Hanfmann and G. Walker. Cambridge, Mass.: MIT Press.

Wason, P. C. (1960). "On the failure to eliminate hypotheses in a conceptual task." *Quarterly Journal of Experimental Psychology* 32: 109–123.

Wason, P. C., and D. Shapiro (1971). "Natural and contrived experience in a reasoning problem." *Quarterly Journal of Experimental Psychology* 23: 63–71.

Wells, M., D. Hestenes, and G. Swackhammer (1995). "A modeling method for high school physics instruction." *American Journal of Physics* 63 (7): 606–619.

Wexler, M., and J. J. A. van Boxtel (2005). "Depth perception by the active observer." *Trends in Cognitive Science* 9: 431–438.

Wexler, M., S. M. Kosslyn, and A. Berthoz (1998). "Motor processes in mental rotation." *Cognition* 68: 77–94.

Wilson, D. (1983). *Rutherford: Simple Genius*. London: Hodder and Stoughton.

Wise, N. (1979). "The mutual embrace of electricity and magnetism." *Science* 203: 1313–1318.

Wiser, M. (1995). "Use of history of science to understand and remedy students' misconceptions about time and temperature." In *Software Goes to School*, 23–38, ed. D. Perkins. New York, Oxford University Press.

Wohlschlager, A. (2001). "Mental object rotation and the planning of hand movements." *Perception and Psychophysics* 63 (4): 709–718.

Woods, D. D. (1997). "Towards a theoretical base for representation design in the computer medium: Ecological perception and aiding human cognition." In *The Ecology of Human–Machine Systems*, 157–188, ed. J. Flach, P. Hancock, J. Caird, and K. Vincente. Hillsdale, N.J.: Lawrence Erlbaum.

Yaner, P. W. (2007). "From shape to function: Acquisition of teleological models from design drawings by compositional analogy." College of Computing. Atlanta, GA, Georgia Institute of Technology. Doctoral dissertation.

Yeh, W., and L. W. Barsalou (1996). "The role of situations in concept learning." In *Proceedings of the Cognitive Science Society 18*, 469–474, ed. G. W. Cottrell. Hillsdale, N.J.: Lawrence Erlbaum.

Zhang, J. (1997). "The nature of external representations in problem solving." *Cognitive Science* 21 (2): 179–217.

Zhang, J., and D. A. Norman (1995). "A representational analysis of numeration systems." *Cognition* 57: 271–295.

Zwaan, R. A. (1999). "Situation models: The mental leap into imagined worlds." *Current Directions in Psychological Science* 8: 15–18.

Zwaan, R. A., and G. A. Radvansky (1998). "Situation models in language comprehension and memory." *Psychological Bulletin* 123: 162–185.

Index

Spatial simulation, mental, 110–112
Spirals, 77, 78
Spring(s). *See also* Rod-spring model
  concept of, 65–67
  torsion, S2, and, 186
Static electricity, 43–44
Steiner, Mark, 49
Stress tensor, 34
Structural alignment and projection,
  syntactic theory of, 149–150
Structural consistency, 148–149
Structural focus, 148
Sundevall, G., 188–189
Symbol grounding problem, 124
Symbol system, physical, 96
Symmetry argument vs. Maxwell's
  modeling, 48–52
Syntactic theory of structural align-
  ment and projection, 149–150
Systematicity, 149

Tao, Terrance, 91, 216n13
Thagard, Paul, 150
Think-aloud protocol, 63. *See also* S2
Thomson, W., 22, 27–30, 51
Thought-experimental narratives,
  173–180
Topological transformations, 72, 88
Torsion, 15, 83, 89, 186
  recognizing, 141–143, 167–170
  sequence of generic transformation in
    discovering, 89, 90
Transfer and mapping. *See* Mapping
  and transfer
Transformations, types of, 111
Translational motion, 37–38

Verbal analysis, 64–65
Vortex fluid, 29–35
Vortex–idle wheel, 35–44. *See also under*
  Maxwell
  elastic, 44–48
Vygotsky, Lev Semyonovich, 183

Wason card task, 102
Wise, Norton, 26–27
Wittgenstein, Ludwig, 91
Working memory representations, 99,
  108, 121, 125

Zigzag wire, 73–75

Printed in the United States
By Bookmasters